A Multidisciplinary Handbook

of Child and Adolescent
Mental Health for
Front-line Professionals

of related interest

Mental Health Interventions and Services for Vulnerable Children and Young People
Edited by Panos Vostanis
Foreword by Richard Williams
ISBN 978 1 84310 489 6

Introducing Mental Health
A Practical Guide
Caroline Kinsella and Connor Kinsella
Foreword by Vikram Patel
ISBN 978 1 84310 260 1

Cool Connections with Cognitive Behavioural Therapy
Encouraging Self-esteem, Resilience and Well-being in Children and Young People Using CBT Approaches
Laurie Seiler
ISBN 978 1 84310 618 0

By Their Own Young Hand
Deliberate Self-harm and Suicidal Ideas in Adolescents
Keith Hawton and Karen Rodham with Emma Evans
ISBN 978 1 84310 230 4

Understanding Attachment and Attachment Disorders
Theory, Evidence and Practice
Vivien Prior and Danya Glaser
ISBN 978 1 84310 245 8

Children with Mental Disorder and the Law
A Guide to Law and Practice
Anthony Harbour
ISBN 978 1 84310 576 3

The Complete Guide to Asperger's Syndrome
Tony Attwood
ISBN 978 1 84310 495 7 (hardback)
ISBN 978 1 84310 669 2 (paperback)

A Multidisciplinary Handbook

# of Child and Adolescent Mental Health for Front-line Professionals

Second Edition

Nisha Dogra, Andrew Parkin,
Fiona Gale and Clay Frake

Foreword by Panos Vostanis

Jessica Kingsley Publishers
London and Philadelphia

First edition published in 2002

This edition published in 2009
by Jessica Kingsley Publishers
116 Pentonville Road
London N1 9JB, UK
and
400 Market Street, Suite 400
Philadelphia, PA 19106, USA

www.jkp.com

Library of Congress Cataloging in Publication Data
A multidisciplinary handbook of child and adolescent mental health for front-line professionals / Nisha Dogra ... [et al.] ; foreword by Panos Vostanis. -- 2nd ed.
p. ; cm.
Includes bibliographical references and index.
ISBN 978-1-84310-644-9 (pbk. : alk. paper) 1. Child mental health--Handbooks, manuals, etc. 2. Adolescent psychology--Handbooks, manuals, etc. 3. Child mental health services--Handbooks, manuals, etc. I. Dogra, Nisha, 1963-
[DNLM: 1. Mental Health. 2. Adolescent Psychology. 3. Child Psychology. 4. Mental Health Services. WS 105.5.M3 M961 2008]
RJ499.3.M855 2008
618.92'89--dc22

2008013295s

British Library Cataloguing in Publication Data
A CIP catalogue record for this book is available from the British Library

ISBN 978 1 84310 644 9

Printed and bound in Great Britain by
Athenaeum Press, Gateshead, Tyne and Wear

Contents

Part 5: Treatment and Management Strategies

Part 6: Medico-Legal Aspects of Child Mental Health

Part 7: Exercise and Case Study Solutions

List of Tables

List of Figures

Foreword

Child mental health services are rapidly expanding around the world, albeit at different paces and through different models and systems. Policies and legislation in recent years have created a favourable framework for services to develop, in particular through inter-agency working. It is thus widely accepted that all agencies have an important role to play in enhancing children's mental health. Developing professional skills and improving the workforce across different agency domains is, therefore, a major challenge in delivering high quality services for children, young people and their families.

The second edition of *A Multidisciplinary Handbook of Child and Adolescent Mental Health* is nicely positioned within this context of establishing a common 'service language' on child mental health concepts, assessments and interventions. The authors have successfully integrated key research findings and practice messages that apply across organisations and practitioner groups routinely involved in children's welfare.

The updated text incorporates recent evidence-base and guidelines for interventions on common behavioural, emotional and developmental problems in childhood and young life, with extended information on topics such as self-harm and cultural diversity. The structure, format and friendly writing style convey the key messages, and these are integrated with case material within front-line professionals' and agencies' remits. In that respect, this textbook will be of interest and value to a range of practitioners, as well as students and parents or carers, and will serve as foundation to child mental health training programmes. Its implications go beyond any particular country or system of children's services provision.

Panos Vostanis
Professor of Child Psychiatry
University of Leicester

Acknowledgements

All the authors would like to thank the following colleagues who have in one way or another provided constructive criticism or comments to support the writing of this book: Dr Karen Bretherton, who contributed to the learning disability part in the original text; Professor Vostanis for the foreword and a special thank you to the artists who contributed to this book: Ashwynn Dhar, Priya Dhar, Rebecca Frake and Michael Frake whose drawings are used throughout this edition.

Finally we would like to thank all our families, friends and colleagues who provided support in their different ways.

How to Get the Best Out of this Handbook

This handbook aims to:

- provide an introduction to child mental health
- raise key issues in this field.

This handbook may be used for:

- raising awareness of child mental health
- acquiring a basic grounding in child mental health
- supporting staff who deal with child mental health problems in a non-health context at all levels
- supporting staff who deal with child mental health problems in primary health care
- supporting mental health specialists who engage in training professionals about child mental health.

Structure of the book

Part 1: Defining and meeting the mental health needs of children and young people

This part begins by considering the definition of mental health and the stigmatisation around mental health issues. It then reviews service organisation and provision of services to meet young people's mental health needs before considering assessment of mental health at different levels. Interviewing young people and their families as well as the contents of specialist mental health assessment are outlined.

Part 2: Child and family development

This part is designed to cover all aspects of child, adolescent and family development and their relationship and impact on mental health. The emphasis is on a sound theoretical knowledge of *normal* development. Clinical examples are used to illustrate the theory and help the reader relate it to their own practice.

Part 3: Factors that influence the mental health of young people

This part discusses the factors that play a part in the causation of mental health problems in young people. It also considers the predisposing, precipitating and perpetuating factors that impact on child mental health in addition to considering wider influences. Protective and adverse factors are highlighted. It also considers young people in vulnerable groups at high risk of developing mental health problems.

Part 4: Specific mental health problems of childhood and adolescence

This part details the group of mental health problems that can occur in infancy, childhood and adolescence, and considers specific common disorders/problems.

When describing disorders we have provided information on presentation, risk factors, assessment and management. When the principles of a group of disorders are very similar we have combined features to prevent needless repetition.

Part 5: Treatment and management strategies

This part is designed to cover the key principles and strategies in the management of child mental health problems. There is an overview of strategies available with an emphasis on planning management with effective resource use. We have discussed a range of options and highlighted those that are particularly appropriate to use at primary care level.

Part 6: Medico–legal aspects of child mental health

This part highlights the key legislation that relates to children and mental health including the Human Rights Act, the Children Act and the Mental Health Act.

Part 7: Exercise and case study solutions

We have tried to make this book as interactive as possible and hope that you will find the exercises and case studies that appear throughout useful and enjoyable. The final part provides possible solutions to the case studies and some of the exercises that appear throughout the book. There are of course a range of issues and permutations, but in providing solutions we have tried to focus on key issues.

Introduction to terms used in the book

To try to avoid clumsy sentences we have used terms in the following ways as a form of shorthand and convenience, rather than to imply that any one term is better than, or preferred to, another.

We have used the term *young people* when we are talking about children and adolescents up until the age of 18. Where we are specifically referring to under fives we have used the term *preschool children*. Where we refer to children up to age 12, we have used the word *children*. We have used the term *adolescence* when we are specifically thinking about the developmental aspects of those aged between 13 and 18 years. When talking broadly about the discipline of *child mental health* we have used this term as it stands (rather than refer to the mental health of young people), given that it remains a widely used and accepted term. The same applies to *child psychiatry* and derivatives thereof.

When we have referred to a *parent–child* relationship we have used the term irrespective of the young person's age as it is the relationship that is of relevance. We have used the term *parents* instead of parents/carers/guardians. Where we have stated parents, it could easily read carers or guardians or indeed the singular of any of these but again we wanted to avoid wordiness by trying to cover all possibilities. This does not apply in the section related to attachment where the term *primary attachment figure* has been used as it applies to a specific context.

Again as shorthand we have used the *family* and this term includes the biological family and parts thereof, step, foster, adoptive and other types of families. We have used the term *staff in primary care* to include healthcare, education, social services and voluntary agency staff rather than calling it tier one as the Health Advisory Service Report is applicable to England and Wales only.

The term *professional* has been used throughout the book and refers to anyone who works with young people, whether in the primary care level or within specialist services. We have avoided the use of the word clinical as many primary care level professionals do not have a clinical remit or responsibility.

The term *disorder* is used when we are talking about severe and clearly specified mental health problems. In all other situations we refer to *mental health problems*. As this book is written for a wide audience we have either avoided the use of specialist language or we have defined it.

To avoid overwhelming readers with detailed referencing we have given references for key theories only, instead providing a wide reading list. Some of the texts are very specialist but may be useful for some readers, depending on their role.

Abbreviations

ADD   attention deficit disorder

ADHD   attention deficit hyperactivity disorder

CAMHS   child and adolescent mental health service or services

DSM   American Psychiatric Association (2000) *Diagnostic and Statistical Manual of Mental Disorders* (4th edition). Text Revision (DSM-IV-TR). Arlington, VA: American Psychiatric Association.

EWO   educational welfare officer

GP   general practitioner

HAS   Health Advisory Service

HRA   Human Rights Act 1998

ICD   *WHO (1992) The International Classification of Diseases, ICD-10 Classification of Mental and Behavioural Disorders.* Geneva: World Health Organization.

MHA   Mental Health Act

OCD   obsessive-compulsive disorder

PCMHW primary child mental health worker

PDD   pervasive developmental disorder

SSRI   selective serotonin reuptake inhibitor

WHO   World Health Organization

PART 1

Defining and Meeting the Mental Health Needs of Children and Young People

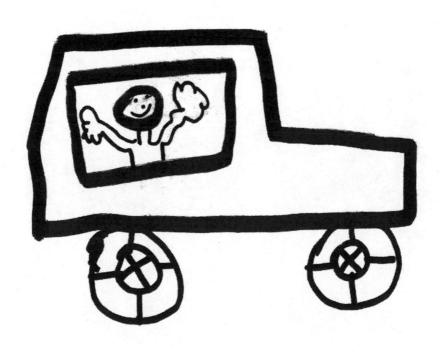

CHAPTER 1

Defining Mental Health

Definitions of mental health

The Health Advisory Service Report (HAS Report 1995) *Together We Stand* defined mental health in children and young people as:

- a capacity to enter into and sustain mutually satisfying personal relationships

- continuing progression of psychological development

- an ability to play and learn so that attainments are appropriate for age and intellectual level

- a developing moral sense of right and wrong

- not necessarily present when psychological distress or maladaptive behaviour is appropriate given a child's age or context.

This definition implies that there is an ideal state of mental health that all strive to reach. Another similar and also commonly used definition (Mental Health Foundation 1999) states that children who are emotionally healthy will have the ability to:

- develop psychologically, emotionally, creatively, intellectually and spiritually

- initiate, develop and sustain mutually satisfying personal relationships

- use and enjoy solitude

- become aware of others and empathise with them

- play and learn

- develop a sense of right and wrong
- resolve (face) problems and setbacks and learn from them.

Again this definition may be criticised for presenting an idealised and simplified view of mental health. It also perhaps fails to acknowledge the diversity of human responses to different experiences and the diversity of human individuality and ability. However, both definitions focus on trying to define what mentally healthy young people should be able to do should they so wish, and in that way they begin to provide some clarity about when young people are not mentally healthy. The second definition also makes no mention of the impact of developmental issues playing a central part when considering young people's mental health.

Mental health is to some extent a culturally bound concept, and these definitions are clearly set out from Western perspectives. Despite this, they provide a common starting point from which young people's mental health can be considered. It is important to remember that good mental health is not a static state, good mental health is dependent on several factors and a change in these factors may lead to changes in mental health status. The World Health Organization (WHO) (2001) states that mental health is an integral component of health through which a person realises his or her own cognitive, affective and relational abilities. With a balanced mental disposition, one is more effective in coping with the stresses of life, can work productively and fruitfully, and is able to make a positive contribution to one's community. Mental disorders affect mental health and impede or diminish the possibility of reaching all or part of the goals above.

It is important to emphasise that there is a continuum between emotional and mental well-being and mental disorder or mental illness. At one end of the spectrum is complete mental health and at the other severe mental disorder. The continuum between the range of 'normal' human experience and mental disorder (with the exception of psychosis) means that the cut-off between what is normal and abnormal can be hard to define. It is not just the presence of symptoms that defines a disorder but also its impact on the individual's functioning. For example, feelings of anxiety before big events are perceived as a normal response and something that most people experience. However, in some individuals the levels of anxiety may prevent functioning and therefore warrant attention. In others the symptoms may be severe but manageable and therefore not seen as limiting. Similarly, a phobia of spiders may have little impact on an individual, whereas a phobia of needles may be less easily ignored.

Using the notion of a continuum, there are behaviours which in certain contexts *may* indicate mental illness. These include erratic behaviour; mood lability (changeable mood); agitation; disinhibition; paranoia; incoherent speech; unusual or inappropriate behaviour; repetitive actions; hearing voices; and holding fixed irrational beliefs that are not culturally contextual. However, it is important to note that these behaviours may also be indicative of other problems that are not associated with mental health.

There can be an inability or unwillingness by some young people, parents and professionals to recognise that distress is a component of human experience and not necessarily a mental health problem. If this is recognised, it can be appropriately addressed rather than labelled as a mental health problem and passed on to specialists for management. It is also important to empower individuals to take responsibility for their own health, including mental health, in appropriate ways. That requires greater openness and willingness to talk about mental health. It means making mental health everyone's business. All professionals working with young people have a responsibility to consider young people's psychological health as well as to pay attention to their physical health.

Stigmatisation

The severe and pervasive effects of the stigma of mental health are known to impact on individuals and families, and can result in intense feelings of shame, social exclusion and a reluctance to seek help (Wahl 1999). There is an increasing body of knowledge that explores the impact of stigma in children and young people, who may have mental health needs. There is potential for the effects of stigma to be so insidious that it can significantly reduce access to children's mental health services; it can create fear, marginalisation and low self-esteem in children, and diminish the effectiveness of interventions. Stigma can have such a significant effect that there is a potential for mental health problems to increase in severity. Often, the experience of stigma has been described as on a par with the experience of having a mental health problem (Gale 2008).

Many of the terms used to describe individuals with mental health problems are derogatory. Individuals with mental illness are often perceived to be unpredictable (volatile, emotional, unstable, off the wall), aggressive (violent, crazy) or having something missing (a slice short of a loaf; a penny short of a pound; lights are on but no one's home; etc.). There is little differentiation between mental health problems and formal mental illness. Terms may be loosely used and poorly understood. There is also a discrepancy between lay and professional use of widely used terms such as depression, panic and stress.

Stigmatisation is a worldwide phenomenon as shown by the need for the five-year anti-stigma campaign 'Changing minds – Every family in the land', which began in the UK in 1998 (Royal College of Psychiatrists 1998), and by the WHO campaign 'Stop exclusion – Dare to care' (WHO 2001). There is still much to be done in reducing the stigma attached to mental health problems by individuals and organisations. Mental health problems are stigmatised by health professionals and the public alike, although the degrees may vary. There are at least two main reasons for stigmatisation, which is a complex area. The first is fears regarding people with mental health problems because of perceived aggression and unpredictability; there can also be fears that individuals with mental illness have criminal intentions. The second relates to concerns that there can be a fine line between 'normal' experience and mental health problems. It is often easier to see mental health problems as belonging to others (i.e. the 'them-and-us' mentality) as this allows individuals not to have to consider the vulnerability we all have to experiencing mental health problems. A fear of the unknown and an unwillingness to be open about mental illness can perpetuate prejudice.

Negative attitudes towards the subject of mental health problems and those who experience mental health problems are already present in young people with beliefs that little can be done to address the problems of stigmatisation (Bailey 1999). When attempts are made to address stigmatisation of mental health, interventions need to be made at all levels, i.e. with individuals, with communities, with institutions and at strategic and policy making level. There is a tendency to avoid using terms such as 'mental health' and an emerging preference to talk about 'emotional literacy' or 'positive health' thus colluding with the assumption that 'mental' is a negative and pejorative term. Experience shows that the attitudes of mental health professionals can help shape attitudes towards those with mental health problems. Therefore those working in the mental health field need to ensure that they do not subconsciously change their language to accommodate prejudice.

Exercise 1.1

1. How comfortable are you talking about mental health and mental health problems?

2. What terms do you use to describe mental health problems or individuals experiencing mental health problems?

3. What is your own understanding and experience of mental health and mental health problems?

4. Do you think there are areas of your practice in which you could do more to help destigmatise mental health problems? If not, what are you already doing to ensure that you provide equitable services (whatever area you are in) to all young people you come into contact with?

5. If you think you could do more to destigmatise mental health, how do you think you might be able to do this?

References
Bailey, S. (1999) 'Young people, mental illness and stigmatisation.' *Psychiatric Bulletin 23*, 107–110.

Gale, F. (2008) 'Tackling the stigma of mental health in vulnerable children and young people.' In P. Vostanis (ed.) *Mental Health Interventions and Services for Vulnerable Children and Young People.* London: Jessica Kingsley Publishers.

Health Advisory Service Report (1995) *Together We Stand: The Commissioning, Role and Management of Child and Adolescent Mental Health Services.* London: HMSO.

Mental Health Foundation (1999) *Bright Futures: Promoting Children and Young People's Mental Health.* London: Mental Health Foundation.

Royal College of Psychiatrists (1998) *Changing Minds: Every Family in the Land. Recommendations for the implementation of a five year strategy 1998–2003.* London: Royal College of Psychiatrists.

Wahl, O.F. (1999) 'Mental health consumers' experience of stigma.' *Schizophrenia Bulletin 25*, 467–478.

World Health Organization (2001) *World Health Day. Mental Health: Stop Exclusion – Dare to Care.* Available at www.who.int/world-health-day/previous/2001/files/whd2001_dare_to_care_en.pdf, accessed on 18 July 2008.

Further reading
Armstrong, C. (2000) 'Young people's perceptions of mental health.' *Children and Society 14*, 60–72.

Armstrong, C., Hill, M. and Secker, J. (1998) *Listening to Children.* London: Mental Health Foundation.

Spitzer, A. and Cameron, C. (1995) 'School-age children's perceptions of mental illness.' *Weston Journal of Nursing Research 17*, 4, 398–415.

Vostanis, P. (ed.) (2007) *Mental Health Interventions and Services for Vulnerable Children and Young People.* London: Jessica Kingsley Publishers.

Weiss, M.F. (1994) 'Children's attitudes toward the mentally ill: An eight-year longitudinal follow-up.' *Psychology Reports 74*, 51–56.

CHAPTER 2

Meeting the Mental Health Needs of Young People

How common are mental health problems in young people?

It is now recognised that many mental health problems can begin in childhood. Given the number of epidemiological studies (surveys that are usually based in the community and aim to identify the number of individuals experiencing specific problems), it can be somewhat difficult to understand why there are still such variable rates of recorded prevalence (that is the number of cases) of mental health problems in young people. Generally studies use one of two approaches. The first is to use the classification and diagnostic manuals that exist – the *Diagnostic and Statistical Manual of Mental Disorders* (American Psychiatric Association 2000) and the *International Classification of Diseases* (WHO 1992). A disorder is classed as present if the diagnostic criteria are met as defined by these manuals. The second approach is to ask about general symptomatology and describe 'caseness' (that is that the person being asked has enough symptoms to be defined as a clinical case) if a certain threshold is reached irrespective of what the diagnosis is on a classificatory system.

Studies will give different results depending on the measures used and the cultural context in which they are used. The Child Behaviour Checklist (CBCL: Achenbach and Edelbrock 1983) is a widely-used measure and has been developed to be completed by parents, young people and teachers. It defines caseness by a checklist, which is then scored. A prevalence study using the CBCL in Vietnam found that Vietnamese young people had lower CBCL scores than standard US norms (McKelvey *et al.* 1999).

This may reflect a true difference in the prevalence of disorders or it may reflect different cultural conceptualisation of what constitutes a disorder or a problem. The design of the measure may also be culturally contextual.

The World Health Organization (2001) states that approximately one in five of the world's youth (15 years and younger) suffer from mild to severe disorders and that a large number of these young people remain untreated as services simply do not exist. Other figures given by WHO support the view that young people's mental health is an important issue: for example 17 million young people aged 5–17 in Latin America and the Caribbean are affected by disorders severe enough to require treatment; 10 per cent of schoolchildren in Alexandria, Egypt, suffer from depression, and anxiety in final-year schoolchildren is 17 per cent. In the US an estimated one in ten young people have mental illness severe enough to cause some level of impairment, but less than 20 per cent of those needing treatment receive it (National Institute of Mental Health 2000). A UK survey (Office for National Statistics 2005) found rates of 10 per cent in 5–15-year-olds of similar mental health disorders. Generally the cross-cultural comparison tends to show that there are great similarities in the characteristics of psychopathology manifested in different settings although rates of symptomatology vary (Bird 1996). Prevalence rates of child mental health problems are generally between 15 and 20 per cent. The diagnostic measure studies are less comparable than the ones using CBCL as they have a greater potential for different interpretations. However, it is still difficult to say whether the divergent rates reflect different rates in different cultures or contexts or differing data collection methods.

There also different rates between the same population who live in different environments. The prevalence rates for inner-city areas are generally higher than for rural areas. The prevalence rates using diagnostic measures range from 12.4 per cent (in France) to 51.3 per cent (in Germany) but are consistently above 10 per cent. Even studies that have different prevalence figures consistently show that boys have greater rates of 'externalising' problems (i.e. problems that are expressed through behaviour that impacts on the external environment, such as aggression, non-compliance, and so on) and girls of 'internalising' problems (i.e. behaviours that reflect a turning inwards, such as depression, anxiety and deliberate self-harm) (Bird 1996). Prepubertal girls have fewer problems than boys of the same age, but the rates of problems in girls increase with age. Rates are also consistently higher in poorer deprived areas. Rates also vary between reports by parents and self-reports by young people.

Levels of service provision

The HAS Report (1995) suggested a four-tier model and, in the UK, this has become widely accepted although the definition of the tiers is not always clear. While the definitions for tier one and four are usually consistently used, those for tiers two and three are less clear.

Tier one

This tier describes agencies that offer first-line services to the public and with whom they make direct contact. It encompasses education, social services, health and voluntary agencies. This level is beyond that of the support available within the family and community and involves outside agencies in the management of the young person's problems. Tier one services are also often referred to as universal services. These are services (sometimes also referred to as mainstream services) that are provided to, or are routinely available to, all children and their families. Universal services are designed to meet the sorts of needs that all children have; they include early years provision, mainstream schools and youth services for example, as well as health services provided by GPs, midwives, and health visitors.

At tier one there may also be targeted services that provide support aimed at particular groups of children, but often from within universal (or mainstream) services. This includes services such as Sure Start Children's Centres that are aimed at all children in a targeted area where children are known to be less likely to achieve optimal outcomes. It also includes services provided directly to individual children who have been identified as having additional needs, such as those provided via schools to children with special educational needs. Targeted services also include services aimed at groups of children and their families with complex needs, such as targeted parenting support (Every Child Matters 2003). This document also states that 'Embedding targeted services within universal settings can ensure more rapid support without the delay of formal referral, and enable frontline practitioners to seek help and advice. Developing networks across universal and specialist professionals can strengthen inter-professional relationships and trust' (Every Child Matters 2003, p.63). It is difficult to be sure that this is the case in practice.

Tier two

This is defined as healthcare provided in the health service by individuals from a variety of multidisciplinary backgrounds. Traditionally, these individuals are psychiatrists, psychologists, psychiatric nurses, occupational therapists, psychotherapists and social workers. Tier two could include those primary level staff in health, social services, education, specialist voluntary agencies or non-governmental organisations who have specialist training or responsibilities relating to mental health.

Tier three

This is defined as the working together of different members of the multidisciplinary team who also provide tier two care. It is this issue that has led to some confusion. Resources alone may determine whether one or two members of the multidisciplinary team work together. Tiers two and three are made up of the same professionals, but the tier they are placed in at any point in time is defined by their working practice on a particular case. For the purposes of this book, tiers two and three will be combined, as from a tier one perspective the distinction between the tiers is less important than the need for specialist mental health services.

Tier three also includes more detailed multidisciplinary assessments of individuals over a longer period of time than is usual for tier two. This includes day resource assessment and management facilities, which use the input from all members of a multidisciplinary team to provide different perspectives. They usually see young people who have been seen by tier two/three staff in an outpatient clinic context.

Tier four

This is defined as very specialised interventions and care provided by health, social and education services for relatively few, but very troubled, young people who have complex psychological and psychiatric problems. It includes inpatient services as well as regional and national centres that provide specific interventions. However, young people may need access to inpatient care for their mental health needs without the involvement of other agencies. The healthcare staff though will need to liaise with education services to ensure that the young person's educational needs are met.

Whatever the criticism of the HAS Report model, it has proved to be useful to help conceptualise and plan young people's mental health services from prevention through to the management of mental health problems.

The management of young people's mental health problems in primary care
Introduction

For many young people, especially preschool children, attendance at the General Practitioner's (GP or family doctor) service is very common. On average around 90 per cent of preschool children are taken to their GP in one year. This figure is still high among older children, around 65 per cent per year. Although the majority of young people see their doctor for physical health problems, a small proportion (2–5%) present with some form of mental health problem (emotional or behavioural difficulties). In recent studies of attenders at GP surgeries, one in four children aged 7–12 years were found to have mental health problems and four in ten amongst 13–16-year-olds (Kramer and Garralda 2000). These rates are higher than those found in the general community.

A range of mental health problems is seen in primary care. These problems can include behavioural problems, hyperactivity and anxiety, all of which can cause major concerns for parents. There can also be an increased presentation of young people suffering from mental health problems with up to a quarter of children attending with associated physical symptoms (such as headaches, nausea, abdominal pain). These presentations are sometimes called psychosomatic presentations – that is, physical symptoms are presented but the underlying problem is psychological.

Although the figures relate to known presentations, it is acknowledged that many more problems are present in the general population that are either not recognised or not presented. Professionals in primary care are well positioned to recognise and to provide assessment and treatment for emerging mental health problems in young people, whilst identifying those who require intervention from specialist child and adolescent mental health services (CAMHS). They are also well placed to develop and contribute to preventive strategies concerning young people's mental health.

Voluntary sector/other community professionals/ non-governmental organisations (local and others)

- Home Start
- family service units
- SureStart
- Barnardo's
- National Society for the Prevention of Cruelty to Children (NSPCC)
- Cruse and other bereavement services
- domestic violence projects
- Victim Support and the police
- minority ethnic group projects
- local support groups
- youth workers
- local religious or community leaders
- Red Cross

Health professionals

- general practitioner/ family doctor
- health visitors (including specialist health visitors)
- school nurses
- practice nurses
- district nurses
- midwives
- hospital staff (especially accident and emergency)
- community paediatricians and school doctors

Primary care professionals

Social services

- social workers
- specialist nursery workers
- fostering and adoption staff
- residential social workers
- child protection staff
- youth offending teams
- specialist social work teams, i.e. those working in post-abuse services

Education professionals

- preschool staff
- teachers; special educational needs coordinators (SENCOs)
- educational psychologists
- education welfare officers
- behaviour support staff
- counsellors

Figure 2.1 Primary care professionals — who are they?

Who are the primary care professionals?

The term 'primary care professional' includes any professional who works with young people and is likely to come across their mental health problems first – that is, they are working in the front line with young people and their families. Figure 2.1 illustrates the range of professionals this can include.

The lists of professionals in Figure 2.1 are not comprehensive, but seek to provide an overview of the range and magnitude of professionals working with young people who may encounter and identify mental health problems. Compiling such lists within the local area can be the first step in acknowledging that children's mental health is a universal concern and is therefore 'everyone's business'. Many of the professionals in primary care are able to provide intervention to young people with mental health problems, but staff or their employing organisation may not acknowledge this. It is not always necessary to refer every young person with a mental health problem to a CAMHS. Those that are less disturbed or have their problems identified early may be most appropriately seen and dealt with by primary care.

Interventions in primary care
Information, support and advice

Primary care professionals are in a prime position to provide families with information, support and advice regarding young people's mental health problems and also to implement preventive measures. Simple practices can be useful, such as a range of quality leaflets available for parents regarding specific problems or disorders, or being able to direct people to places where they may obtain information (e.g. local groups or libraries). It is also helpful to have some knowledge of local services available to families; often voluntary action groups, social services or CAMHS may have readily available directories.

Screening and assessment

The key to identification of those young people who require assessment and treatment by specialist CAMHS lies in primary care. Primary care professionals should know what information they need to make an informed decision regarding a young person's mental health. This enables them to manage the problem in primary care or to refer to specialist services as appropriate.

Background information

- name of young person
- consent of parent or person with parental responsibility (i.e. person who is legally recognised as having a responsibility towards the young person), or consent of young person if applicable
- date of birth
- gender
- general practitioner's name
- home address
- the name and address of parents (if different from above)
- ethnic background
- language spoken
- family structure
- is the child in foster care or other substitute care arrangement?
- school – frequency of attendance, whether excluded
- any assessment under the Education Act
- social services involvement (whether there are ongoing child protection investigations/criminal proceedings)
- are there family proceedings for custody/contact or residence in cases of parental separation and divorce?
- other professional involvement (such as private counsellors)

Description of concern in detail

Describe what is happening when and how – getting examples of specific incidents/events may overcome problems of generalisation and jargon in description of behaviour.

- When did it start? (onset)
- How long has it been going on? (duration)
- How often does it happen? (frequency)
- Is it getting worse/remaining the same/getting better?
- What action has been taken to address the concerns by parents and professionals? What has worked so far?
- Are there ongoing medical investigations?
- How is the concern affecting the young person?

Other issues

- physical health
- education*
- social relationships
- activities
- effect on others, i.e. family and significant others
- young person's interests and special talents

---

*   Note: Parental responsibility is defined to include all the rights, powers, authority
    and duties of parents in relation to a child and his or her property.[AQ]

Figure 2.2 Assessment of child mental health problems at primary care level

Many CAMHS offer consultation and training to primary care professionals on child mental health or have key individuals available for the purpose of supporting primary care professionals in their decision-making process. Which professionals can refer to CAMHS is dependent on local arrangements. In some areas only specified professionals can refer directly to CAMHS, whilst other services operate more 'open-door' criteria. When requesting advice on making written referrals to CAMHS in the UK, it is helpful to provide the background information as shown in Figure 2.2. Some services have developed referral forms to help referrers provide the necessary information.

It is important first to obtain valid consent consistent with the referring agency's policy (usually from the parents or legal guardian unless the child is able to consent). However, in some instances consultation can be offered about specific concerns without the need to reveal the identity of the young person or their family.

Direct interventions by primary care professionals

There is a wide range of intervention approaches that primary care professionals can use with young people and their families. It is important to work collaboratively with other agencies, in order to arrange effective programmes of care at an appropriate level.

Interventions can range from preventive work to assessment and treatment of some problems in a variety of settings. Some primary care professionals have developed particular skills in working with young people and families on mental health problems, for example use of behavioural techniques, parenting programmes or development of social skills groups in schools. These are discussed further in Chapter 13.

Exercise 2.1: Personal strengths and skills

Consider what personal strengths and skills you have for working with young people and their families. Then consider which of these skills would benefit from further development and how this would help you fulfil your professional responsibilities.

Consider writing these out and perhaps discussing them with colleagues.

Support for primary care professionals

In the UK, CAMHS have enhanced their support provisions for primary care professionals. Many CAMHS have existing liaison schemes, provided by specialist mental health staff, which offer advice on cases where professionals may be considering a referral to CAMHS. However, following the HAS Report (1995), the primary child mental health worker role has been introduced to complement existing CAMHS provision and further promote mental health service provision in primary care.

What is a primary child mental health worker?

Primary child mental health workers (PCMHW) are CAMHS professionals who work at the interface between primary care and the specialist CAMHS. They can be from a range of backgrounds – registered mental nursing, other areas of nursing (e.g. health visitors), social work, clinical psychology, occupational therapy, or medicine – and should have expertise in working with young people with a range of mental health problems and disorders. Their function is to strengthen and support child and adolescent mental health provision within primary care through direct work with primary care professionals, liaison with primary care staff, consultation and training. The role of PCMHW is very variable in the UK and as yet there is no agreement towards standards such as minimum training and/or qualification requirements. This has perhaps reduced the impact that might have been made.

Exercise 2.2: You and CAMHS

Before reading about specialist CAMHS, consider the following questions:

1. What is your understanding of what a specialist CAMHS does?

2. What is your understanding of the different (clinical) professionals that work within a CAMHS?

3. What are the benefits of primary level staff and CAMHS being aware of each other's role?

4. How might you develop links with your local CAMHS?

Specialist child and adolescent mental health services in the UK

Historically, mental health services for children and young people have been inconsistently organised. The discipline of child psychiatry or child mental health is relatively new, but has a huge variety in the services offered and the way these services are offered. A survey of such services in England and Wales found that they were very patchy, and whilst professionals were committed there was not a real sense of co-ordination or planning (HAS Report 1995). The four-tier model proposed by the HAS Report is one of few models around in terms of planning health provision for young people's mental health needs. Whilst the HAS Report focused on CAMHS in England and Wales, their findings may be applicable to mental health services for young people in other countries.

Whatever models are used, it is widely accepted in the UK that an out-patient service is likely to be suitable for a majority of young people who need specialist services. However, a day resource may also be useful for more detailed assessments and intensive work. In the UK there are very few specialist inpatient child units for mental health problems, and increasingly adolescent inpatient units are being closed. There should be inpatient facilities for mental health disorders of adolescence and it is important these are available within a CAMHS rather than adult service.

The outpatient team should be multidisciplinary. There has sometimes been an assumption that all members of the team serve the same function and all have equal responsibility. This detracts from the purpose of a multidisciplinary team, which is about bringing different perspectives and skills to ensure a wide range of assessments and treatments can be provided. The standard composition is:

- A child psychiatrist – a medical practitioner who has undertaken specialist training in psychiatry and child psychiatry. The specialist role of the psychiatrist is in assessment, diagnostic skills (including differentiation between physical and psychiatric and psychological presentations of health problems), prescribing medications, and (at time of writing) exercising powers under the mental health legislation.

- Clinical nurse specialists or community psychiatric nurses (CPNs) – these nurses have specialist mental health training, and their role is to assess and provide therapeutic interventions including community support for young people with mental health problems and their families.

- Psychologists – specialist skills are in psychometric testing (measuring cognitive ability) and sociometric testing (exploring personality profiles). Their training provides them with grounding in a wide range of psychological and social theories with a greater understanding of behavioural theories and treatments including cognitive behaviour therapy.

- Occupational therapists – their role can be very varied as they come into child mental health with different levels of experience. Their specialist skill is the assessment and treatment of mental health problems using an activity-based approach.

- Primary child mental health workers – as described previously.

The team may also have other specialist therapists, such as family therapists, music therapists and play therapists, but that can be very variable dependent on local resources.

Social workers had until recently been an integral part of the old-style child guidance clinics, but increasingly in some areas they have been less directly involved as an integral part of CAMHS in the UK. Psychologists are sometimes part of the multidisciplinary team, but sometimes operate outside of it although alongside it. Some members of the team may also have undertaken further training in particular therapies such as cognitive behaviour therapy, family therapy and psychotherapy.

The services offered are correspondingly very variable but it is increasingly recognised that many young people referred to specialist CAMHS could actually be managed in the primary care context. There has been increased funding to develop support services such as child behaviour teams and early response projects. It has also become apparent that considerable training is needed to support primary care staff if they are to address these problems and that CAMHS are ideally placed to provide this support and training.

Outpatient teams generally discuss referrals at a team allocation meeting and prioritise them depending on need. In some services the sheer volume of referrals without expansion of services or support services has led to lengthy waiting lists. Whilst this has been difficult, it has also been an opportunity for CAMHS to review their working practices. Some teams will now operate triage clinics where all appropriate referrals are assessed before prioritisation.

Few CAMHS enable open access by tier-one staff to tier-three and tier-four services. The usual point of entry is at tier two, which acts as a filter to the more specialist services. The rationale behind this is that tier-two staff (working either at tier two or three level) can assess the situation before referral to more intensive assessment or therapies.

Inpatient units exist to provide care for young people who cannot best be managed in the community. This not only depends on the severity of their mental health problems but also on the resources or skills that the community (including their family) has for supporting them. Inpatient facilities often face the dilemma of having to respond to acutely ill young people as well as those with less acute but equally debilitating problems in one unit. The needs of these two groups of young people may be very different and it can be difficult to ensure that both are met. Whilst most professionals would agree with guidelines that young people should be admitted to units specifically for young people whenever possible, in practice young people are still often admitted to less than ideal facilities.

Child mental health services are having to question the efficacy of some of the approaches used and provide evidence that the interventions work. The National Institute for Clinical Excellence and Community

Health Improvement Projects will require more critical approaches than the discipline has been used to.

CAMHS may also have training responsibilities for the various disciplines that work within them.

CAMHS in developing countries

As the mental health needs of young people gain more prominence, developing countries are beginning to consider service development and training. Usually this will be in the context of training those who are already in contact with young people (e.g. community and primary care staff). Besides the HAS model, WHO (2001) quotes some projects in the Middle East which have built on supporting primary care staff to deliver basic mental health services to increase access. There is, however, a recognition that primary care staff need to be adequately trained and supervised for this to work effectively. It is useful for service planners to review other models and consider which model suits the context they are planning services for. Development of these services may not currently be a high priority but can include:

- identifying the local priorities of child and adolescent mental health problems

- assessing the effectiveness of interventions and building in effective audit to monitor the standards of service provision

- training to enhance or develop skills of primary healthcare professionals

- research and/or needs analysis and defining the remit of a child and adolescent mental health service in the context of local need

- integrating new services with existing ones and utilising existing resources effectively

- involving the local staff and community in the development of services.

Local staff should particularly be involved in all aspects of development, as ultimately they will be the ones left with the responsibility of ensuring that successful pilot programmes are translated into long-term changes and policy. Dogra *et al.* (2005) and Omigbodun *et al.* (2007) describe training programmes in India and Nigeria respectively and demonstrate some of the issues discussed above.

Exercise 2.3: Mapping local services

Draw up a list of local resources that you are aware of for addressing the mental health problems of young people and services for parents to enable them to parent and support young people. To your list add the problem or issue that the resource addresses, and how to contact them.

When you read Part 4 it may be useful to repeat this exercise and identify resources to address the problems that you are commonly faced with.

References

Achenbach, T.M. and Edelbrock, C. (1983) *Manual for the Child Behavior Checklist and Revised Child Behavior Profile.* Burlington: University of Vermont.

American Psychiatric Association (2000) *Diagnostic and Statistical Manual of Mental Disorders* (4th edition). Text Revision (DSM-IV-TR). Arlington, VA: American Psychiatric Association.

Bird, H. (1996) 'Epidemiology of childhood disorders in a cross-cultural context.' *Journal of Child Psychology and Psychiatry 37*, 1, 35–49.

Dogra, N., Frake, C., Bretherton, K., Dwivedi, K. and Sharma, I. (2005) 'Training CAMHS professionals in developing countries: An Indian case study.' *Child and Adolescent Mental Health 10*, 2, 74–79.

Every Child Matters (2003) London: The Stationery Office.

Health Advisory Service Report (1995) *Together We Stand: The Commissioning, Role and Management of Child and Adolescent Mental Health Services.* London: HMSO.

Kramer, T. and Garralda, E.M. (2000) 'Child and adolescent mental health problems in primary care.' *Advances in Psychiatric Treatment 6*, 287–294.

McKelvey, R.S., Davies, L.C., Sang, D.L., Pickering, K.R. and Tu, H.C. (1999) 'Problems and competencies reported by parents of Vietnamese children in Hanoi.' *Journal of the American Academy of Child and Adolescent Psychiatry 38*, 6, 731–737.

National Institute of Mental Health (2000) *Treatment of Children with Mental Disorders.* Available at www.nimh.nih.gov/health/publications/treatment-of-children-with-mental-disorders/complete.pdf, accessed on 18 July 2008.

Office for National Statistics (2005) *The Mental Health of Children and YoungPeoplein Great Britain, 2004.* Basingstoke, Palgrave McMillan.

Omigbodun, O., Bella, T., Dogra, N. and Simoyan, O. (2007) 'Training health professionals for child and adolescent mental health care in Nigeria: A qualitative analysis.' *Child and Adolescent Mental Health 12*, 3, 132–137.

World Health Organization (1992) *The International Classification of Diseases, ICD-10 Classification of Mental and Behavioural Disorders.* Geneva: World Health Organization.

World Health Organization (2001) *World Health Day. Mental Health: Stop Exclusion – Dare to Care.* Available at www.who.int/world-health-day/previous/2001/files/whd2001_dare_to_care_en.pdf, accessed on 18 July 2008.

CHAPTER 3

Assessment of Young People's Mental Health

Interviewing young people
Introduction
A successful interview depends on the professional thinking very carefully about appropriate engagement with the young person and family. It is important to outline the proposed structure or plan of the interview and ground rules regarding confidentiality. For younger members of the family it is helpful to explain what is going to happen to dispel any fears or uncertainties, that is it will usually involve talking together and going home at the end of the meeting. Young people and their parents need information about what your service does after introductions have been made. Clarifying the expectations of everyone present assists the assessment process. If the family have concerns or anxieties about seeing you, these need to be addressed. There also needs to be consideration of whether the family is seen together or the young person is seen individually.

Consent
There are governing principles of good clinical practice, which include providing information in an age-appropriate and accessible way to young people. Their views need to be ascertained and clear explanations provided of what is happening. It is worth asking children to explain their understanding so any misunderstandings can be corrected. Children may respond better to communicating their concerns through non-verbal methods.

Although they do not acquire full adult rights to make their own decisions until they are 18, young people in England and Wales aged 16 and 17 are also presumed to be competent to give consent and should be treated as such unless there is evidence to suggest otherwise, such as severe intellectual disability, or temporary inability to consent due to severe mental illness. There is no lower age limit in Scotland. A 16- or 17-year-old only needs to be 'capable of expressing his own wishes'.

An expert government committee has suggested that the presumption of competence to consent should arise at around age 10 or 12. This may be more appropriate in some conditions than others. Whilst younger children may not be in the position of giving informed consent, it is still important to seek their views as they may have fears or worries which, if addressed, could improve compliance. Consent to healthcare assessments and interventions for people under 16 years of age is normally obtained from parents and the young person's wishes are, where possible, taken into account. Parents usually make appropriate decisions for their children and give consent for treatment on their behalf.

In child mental health, any therapeutic input is limited unless the young person is engaged in the work. It is therefore often useful to engage with the family to explore some of the issues around what they find difficult. However, there may be instances where the young person wishes to consent but does not wish the parents to be involved (and professional opinion respects this wish), or the parents are unavailable or decline or are unable to consent. It is good practice to involve parents or caregivers unless there is a compelling reason not to do so. In such instances, and where assessment or intervention is desirable, the young person should first be assessed as to whether they have the capacity to consent. This is known as 'Gillick competence' – a shorthand way of referring to the landmark judgement in a legal case in England in the 1980s, which ultimately stated that 'the parent's right yields to the child's right to make his own decision as he reaches sufficient understanding and intelligence'. This is a developmental concept and does not fluctuate from day to day but can be developed over time. A judgement about a young person's competence to consent would have to be reconsidered for each different treatment. Whilst there is no lower age limit to Gillick competence, it would be unusual for a child under 12 years to be Gillick competent. The 'Fraser Guidelines' (named after the Law Lord making the judgement) refer specifically to the area of sexual health advice, which was the medical issue in the Gillick case, and have been taken as a guide for all health professionals, not just doctors, and in other specialties. Thus, 'Gillick competence' has taken on a more general meaning. In many cases the terms have become inter-changeable.

Useful checklists for consent taking account of factors that can influ-ence capacity to give consent, including stage of development, have been developed (Pearce 1994; Department of Health 2001). A modified version of Pearce's (1994) checklist is shown in Figure 3.1.

Does the young person have a satisfactory understanding of:	**Other factors**
<ul><li>nature of illness?</li><li>own needs and needs of others?</li><li>risks and benefits to treatment?</li><li>own self-concept?</li><li>significance of time (past, present, future)?</li></ul>	<ul><li>Is the parent–child relationship supportive and affectionate?</li><li>Is there trust and confidence in the doctor–patient relationship?</li><li>Whose opinion influences the child, and how?</li><li>How disabling, chronic or life threatening is the illness?</li><li>Is more time/information needed?</li><li>Is a second opinion required?</li></ul>

Figure 3.1 Checklist for assessing capacity to consent

Confidentiality

You must have a clear understanding of your organisation's policies on confidentiality. Young people are entitled to limited confidentiality. What this means is that young people are entitled to confidentiality as long as maintaining it does not put them at risk. Confidentiality is very important to young people and they often want to know how much of what they say to you is going to be repeated to other adults. Start by explaining what information will be passed on to others, what will be recorded in notes and how the notes will be stored. At the beginning establish that any information you receive that raises child protection issues must be reported to adults and colleagues to ensure the safety of the young person and others. Indeed, guidelines from professional bodies are clear that in these situations young people have a right to be protected. Even when a child is judged to be generally able to make their own decisions, in situations where child protection is an issue child protection overrides confidentiality. Promising confidentiality is unhelpful as this is not a promise that professionals can keep. If confidentiality is promised but later broken the child may find it difficult to trust professionals again. If there is a need to break confidentiality, it is important that this is explained to the child and the reasons for breaking it given. It is also important to ensure that the child is not put in the position of having to take responsibility for sharing the information. Even when older children state they do not want action taken, the safety of children who may be at risk needs to be considered. If abuse is an issue it may be useful to have an initial conversation with the local social services department before referring the situation on to them. It will then be up to social services to decide whether further investigation or action needs to be taken.

The interview
THE SETTING
It is sometimes difficult to control where the meeting takes place. However, try to make the venue as welcoming as possible with comfortable and appropriately arranged seating. Toys or games for younger children can often help to break down the barriers of a formal interview. A board and wipe-off markers (or something similar) may be useful so that young people can share their thoughts and feelings knowing that they can wipe things away before they leave the session. If you meet young people regularly in a variety of settings it is useful to carry some of these items with you, as they are not always readily available in clinics or indeed the young person's home.

Try to ensure you sit at the same level as the young person and that you are not towering above them. It is best to sit by the side of the young person rather than opposite them, which can be very intimidating and appear confrontational. Avoid having tables in the seating area unless you need them for activities.

Allow enough time to listen to the concerns and minimise distractions or interruptions. Remaining in control of the interview shows that there is a structure and focus to the process, which can help reduce anxieties.

LENGTH AND FORMAT OF THE SESSION

Some preparation work before the meeting is essential. It is sometimes hard to estimate how long the meeting will take, but having some notion will help to put both the young person and yourself at ease. Young people are able to sense if you are rushed or do not seem relaxed, which might give the impression that you are uninterested or distracted. An average assessment interview in the community setting is likely to be between 30 and 45 minutes and between 60 and 90 minutes in a CAMHS. In either setting, it may take more than one session to complete the assessment.

Let young people know approximately how long they have and what the format of the meeting will be, so they know what to expect. Often, when asked about their expectations, young people will share their anxieties that they would be interrogated. If possible try to tell them what will happen if you plan to meet again. It can be useful to send them a user-friendly leaflet that describes what will happen during the meeting before they come to see you.

SETTING BOUNDARIES

Clarify what is happening, how you are going to work, what you want them to do and what the 'rules' of the meeting are. Some young people may wish to add a few of their own, for example permission for five minutes break when the session is getting difficult for them. Also ensure that the young person is aware that they are able to interrupt to clarify any concerns throughout, and that they will receive feedback at the end of the meeting. If a young person is verbally abusive, it can be helpful to be clear about what is acceptable behaviour. Professionals should not tolerate abuse but need to be aware that sometimes this is a reflection of illness or distress and in such cases needs sensitive handling.

USE OF LANGUAGE

Tailor your language to the young person's level of comprehension and ability. Use clear explanations that can be easily understood. Listen to how the young person speaks and use language that matches theirs. Watch for signs that they have understood you. If they seem to have misunderstood, then look for another way of explaining. Drawings, cartoons or diagrams can be useful ways of engaging young people.

USING INTERPRETERS

Ensure that you check with an adult who knows the young person what the best way of approaching a meeting with a young person who uses languages (including Signing) other than English might be. Establish which language they feel most comfortable with. If you are not certain that a young person or their family can clearly understand the questions due to language or other communication differences you will need to consider the use of an interpreter. This will add considerably to the time needed to conduct the interview. You should meet with the interpreter before the interview, to brief them on the nature of the information you are seeking and afterwards to clarify any issues of understanding including their view on non-verbal communication and, if possible, the cultural context of the discussion.

It is poor practice to ask a young person or any other member of the family to interpret for their parents. This could put the young person in an awkward or even a dangerous position. Interpreting is highly skilled work and given the nuances of language and meaning inherent in a mental health assessment asking a member of the family to take on this role will compromise the quality of the assessment.

CULTURAL CONSIDERATIONS

Beware of applying stereotypes and making assumptions about individuals and their cultures. A suitable definition of culture is that from the Association of American Medical Colleges (AAMC):

> Culture is defined by each person in relationship to the group or groups with whom he or she identifies. An individual's cultural identity may be based on heritage as well as individual circumstances and personal choice. Cultural identity may be affected by such factors as race, ethnicity, age, language, country of origin, acculturation, sexual orientation, gender, socioeconomic status, religious/spiritual beliefs, physical abilities and occupation, among others. These factors may impact behaviours such as communication styles, diet preferences, health beliefs, family roles, lifestyle, rituals and decision-making processes. All of these beliefs and practices, in turn, can influence how patients and heath care professionals perceive health and illness, and how they interact with one another. (AAMC 1999, p.25)

Our justification for using this definition is that it is a patient-centred definition and can be applied to clinical situations. It suggests that individuals draw upon a range of resources, and that, through the interplay of external and internal meanings, they construct a sense of identity and unique culture. It is also useful because it recognises that both patients and professionals bring a complex individual self to the consultation. This definition also allows for children and their parents to understand the origins of their culture independently. Dogra (2007) outlines how to work with children from diverse backgrounds especially when they are vulnerable.

SEEING YOUNG PEOPLE WITHOUT THEIR PARENTS
During assessment and any subsequent work with any young person and their family, consider spending time individually with the young person. Interviewing a young person individually is usually possible from age four onwards. It can be a valuable source of information, as it will inform decisions about the young person's needs and distinguishes the best way to meet them. The decision regarding whether to interview the young person or not will be guided by the young person's developmental level and confidence.

Adolescents should always be offered the opportunity to be seen individually to understand their views of the difficulties and the impact they have on their life. Some professionals prefer to see the adolescent first before seeing the parents or the rest of the family as this can help in engaging with them. The nature of the young person's problem and the expectations that the family has will often influence the decision, for example a young person with anxiety problems may not be willing to be seen alone.

GIVING FEEDBACK
Ask the young person if they agree to you giving feedback to their parents taking into account issues of confidentiality as discussed above. Explain why you have undertaken certain tasks or activities and ensure that you explain any homework tasks to both the young person and their parents. It can sometimes be useful to provide clear written instructions to engage them in tasks between appointments and to summarise meetings.

Principles of interviewing young people

The key to interviewing young people is listening – not just hearing what they say but also how they say it and how they express themselves. Young people can be very perceptive and if they think they are not being actively listened to they may withdraw or not bother to continue. Listening sensitively and attentively to a young person not only ensures a better quality interview but also helps with gaining the young person's trust and building a relationship. Follow the young person's cues and listen to what they feel is important for them, while trying to understand the meaning. Be clear about your understanding of what the young person is saying. This can be achieved by using reflection – reframing in your own words what you think they are trying to say and checking it out with them, or just repeating back what they have said. It can sometimes be helpful to use drawings or toys to help affirm your understanding.

Try to give feelings expressed by the young person a name: acknowledging their feelings with words will help them to build confidence and a language with which to define their feelings. Help young people to understand that they may experience a range of different feelings and that they may not always be mutually exclusive, for example someone being angry with you does not always mean they do not care about you. You may need to make a statement such as: 'Sometimes, people who have been through what you have been through feel quite scared. I wonder if that's something you have felt.' In this way young people have the permission to share feelings they may feel confused or guilty about.

Think about how you listen to people; are you interested in what they have to say or do you find yourself more interested in your own questions or responses? Think about whether you are able to listen to others or whether you often interrupt. Pay attention to whether you feel comfortable in letting the young person lead the discussion for a while or whether you feel you have to steer it. Recognise your strengths and weaknesses, and get comfortable with them before the interview as they can affect your relationship with the young person. Young people can often spot your uncertainties or anxieties a mile off!

Be careful not to recount your own worries; this can often make the young person feel anxious and unheard. It can be useful to recount stories that relate to someone else's problems to help normalise an issue but this needs to be done carefully. Young people like to feel they are being taken seriously, therefore it is not useful to use their comments as a joke or light relief; but that does not mean humour should not be used when appropriate. It is undermining of the young person to dismiss, belittle or trivialise their experiences by making statements such as 'pull yourself together' or 'it's not the end of the world'.

Avoid being judgemental and critical of young people and their families but ensure you meet your professional responsibilities. Convey warmth and sincerity and have an open and approachable manner whilst maintaining professional standards at all times. Be aware of the young person's cultural and social contexts as this may clarify some of the issues.

INTERVIEWING APPROPRIATE TO THE YOUNG PERSON'S AGE AND STAGE OF DEVELOPMENT

- **Birth to 3 years**
The child is largely dependent on their parents and will not have fully developed language skills. Most interviews should be conducted with adults, but it is important to have the child present so you can observe the child's interactions and abilities.

- **3 to 4 years**
Children will have a vocabulary of around 1000–1500 words and should be able to comprehend and answer some questions. At this stage they will understand rewards and praise, and be able to take turns. They may be able to understand some emotions, such as sad, happy or angry, but will need some explanation of more complex emotions.

This age group usually enjoys simple games or drawings. Assessment of development is usually more successful if framed as a game rather than a formal procedure. Creative use of pictures that relate to emotions is useful to elicit feelings from this age group.

- **4 to 5 years**
Children's language now extends to them being able to talk about meanings of words and they are able to follow directions that have more than one part. Their imagination can provide valuable insights into their worlds by allowing them to tell you a story about themselves. Remember though that some stories may be rather extravagant and their concept of time unclear. The use of dolls or puppets can be

fruitful, as the children may shy away from drawing or want you to do it. The activities should be led by the child but actively engaged in by the professional.

- **6 to 8 years**

At this stage children will be able to give you direct accounts of parts of their own history. Children may be enthusiastic to take part but may become easily bored. However, children may have difficulty in understanding, acknowledging or discussing the presenting problem.

The child will often settle down to prepared worksheets and will be able to comprehend techniques such as 'mood scales' or to complete sentences, such as 'One thing that makes me happy is…' or 'A good thing about me is…'. Give plenty of praise and reward completion of activities with short episodes of 'fun play' before moving on to the next task. Techniques like 'family circles' are useful, where the child puts himself or herself in a circle in the middle of a page and then in a series of evenly spaced circles will place family or friends dependent on their significance to them.

- **9 to 10 years**

During this stage, children respond to being given some responsibility and are able to recognise right and wrong and their feelings of guilt. They will also process information and use it in different situations or to plan ahead.

Techniques that look at consequences and benefits to their behaviours can be useful. The use of 'feelings jugs' is a good technique for this age group. The child has a worksheet with a series of empty jugs, which are labelled with an emotion, and they can colour them in to the level they feel they are at.

- **11 to 13 years**

Young people in this age group begin to take on some adult values, whilst sometimes behaving as a child. They may vary immensely in the way they behave. They may be cooperative and communicative at one end of the spectrum and express themselves through anger at the other. At this age some young people will be organised and have a sense of ownership regarding issues relating to themselves. However, some may appear introspective, sulky or withdrawn, especially in communication with adults.

Techniques that are valuable at this stage can range from diary keeping to poetry and stories, and problem solving. A useful way of looking at problem solving can be using comic strips where the young person can define a range of outcomes to different scenarios. Another useful technique is drawing a 'mountain range' in relation to the ups and downs of a problem or again using mood scales.

- **14 years and over**

Young people begin to take more responsibility and to think about the future. They may express concerns or worries about school, friend-ships and relationships and are able to see things from other people's perspectives.

It can be difficult initially to engage young people in this age group; however, presenting them with a range of choices will encourage them to take responsibility and direct the interview to some extent. Activities that look at making changes or coping with situa-tions can be beneficial, for example looking at an issue or problem in the past, present and future and identifying achievable outcomes with the young person.

Exercise 3.1: Potential difficulties when interviewing young people

How would you manage each of the following scenarios?

1. When the young person has difficulty in separating from the parents.

2. When the parents are anxious about the interview.

3. When the young person is the one who makes the decisions in the family.

4. When the young person refuses to cooperate.

5. When the young person or their parents are hostile, rude or aggressive.

To answer these questions you should refer to Figure 3.1 (p.42).

Case study: Tim

Tim is a 15-year-old boy with a three-month history of low mood (feeling sad), poor concentration, poor sleep, tiredness, lack of interest in playing football (he had been on his school team), with deterioration of his schoolwork. His parents felt he was also irritable and argumentative, which he had not been previously. They were also concerned with ideas of hopelessness although he had not considered self-harm.

Tim refuses to accept a referral to CAMHS.

As a primary care worker what strategies would you employ to engage Tim?

Interviewing families

Families are made up of individuals – an obvious truth, but it is this fact that makes interviewing a family so challenging and sometimes leaves the professional and the family overwhelmed. However, it is this same diversity of individuals that makes the family interview such a potentially rich source of information. Family interviews can also provide perspectives that are unobtainable elsewhere as the family together is so much more than the sum of its parts. It is probably safe to assume that there are at least as many agendas as there are people in the room. In this section we are considering a context when a family is seen together for the purpose of an assessment or family meeting to explore family issues rather than a formal family therapy session. The issues outlined are applicable in several situations, although the techniques will not be applicable to meetings such as case conferences, which have a specific and statutory function.

Preparation

A lot of work can be done before the meeting to maximise the use of the time with the family. A good place to start is to consider what different members of the family might want or expect from the meeting. Young people often feel anxious about the meeting and unsure of its purpose. The possibility of seeking help outside of the family may even have been used as a threat by parents in an attempt to improve the situation. Young people, especially adolescents, may perceive a family meeting variously as a punishment, an opportunity for revenge on their parents or simply an excruciatingly embarrassing experience. Siblings of the referred young person may feel puzzled or upset about their inclusion when they feel their sibling has the problem.

Parents may attend a meeting with a strong hypothesis about the nature of the problem and may find it hard to divert from this agenda. A common experience is parents who feel their child has a particular problem, such as attention deficit hyperactivity disorder. They may perceive exploration of other possible explanations of difficult behaviour as a challenge to that hypothesis. This can prove very tricky for primary care staff who might then feel unable to assert any opinion and feel under pressure to refer on. Other common agendas for parents include the wish to be listened to and to get practical advice and help.

Many parents can feel they have failed as carers if their child has developed mental health problems and so experience an undermining of their skills and authority. The route to an assessment and previous experiences with other agencies often shape the expectations of the family. Considering the nature and source of the information might generate some ideas on these influences.

The professional might also find it useful to reflect on their own position before the meeting and consider how their agency influences the nature of the meeting and how the family perceive the professional. The family might see the professional as being so far removed from their own experience that it creates an unhelpful barrier between them, and the opposite can also apply. This does not mean that professionals need to identify with families, but that they should have an awareness of the possible assumptions made about them by the family. The professional in turn will need to be aware of the assumptions they are making about the family based on the information they have.

Convening a family meeting

The professional may be faced with the decision about who to invite to a family meeting and to some extent this will depend on the way the professional is used to working. One way is to invite the household and go from there. Another approach is to issue an open invitation to whoever the family feel might be helpful, although the extra element of uncertainty may add to the professional's anxiety about being overwhelmed. Whatever approach is chosen, studies of parents' experiences of family meetings show that they value being consulted on this issue and that it goes some way to dispel feelings of failure and disempowerment, making collaboration more likely.

Getting fathers to attend can be difficult and may be indicative of differing gender perceptions of the value of helping agencies, differences of views on the severity of the problem, levels of commitment to the emotional well-being of the family or insecurity of employment. The time of day for the meeting has been shown to be helpful in improving attendance of fathers and school-age siblings.

Professionals may consider working with a colleague when meeting a family if they feel they may be overwhelmed by the amount of information generated in a family meeting. This has the added benefit of introducing another perspective and hence another layer of information. However, this needs careful planning to get the most benefit, for example one professional may concentrate on the parental perspective and the other on the children. Alternatively, the plan might be for one to take a less central role and take an overview of what happens in the meeting (i.e. how things are said, how individuals respond, who says what, who takes a lead, who struggles to get heard, and so on), and for the other to concentrate on the content.

Conducting a family meeting

The issues raised earlier with respect to interviewing young people need equal consideration when undertaking a family meeting. A meeting with a family should start with introductions, explanations of roles and a clarification of the purpose of the meeting. The understanding of the purpose of the meeting is likely to vary between family members and the professional.

It may be that different family members feel constrained about what they say in front of each other. The reasons for this can include: parents not feeling it is appropriate to discuss adult issues in the presence of the children, hitherto undisclosed parentage issues, and fear of violence. It is worth considering meeting different combinations of family members, such as parents only, children only, and individual members. If this is your intention, making this clear at the beginning of the initial session can take the pressure off family members disclosing potentially risky material inappropriately. Surveys of parents who have had family meetings suggest that the opportunity to speak openly without the children is often appreciated.

TYPES OF QUESTION

It is not possible to ask a question without its meaning being interpreted at many different levels, and this process is magnified when interviewing a family. For example, a series of questions about a child's behaviour might be seen by a parent as a criticism of their parenting skills and at the same time by the child as the professional taking sides with the parent. At first glance, this realisation might paralyse the professional, but it is helpful to note patterns of questions and answers that might occur in a session. One example is a temptation the professional experiences to direct questions at the most receptive member of the family, which marginalises the more ambivalent, hostile or quiet members and limits the perspectives. It might also negate most of the benefits of interviewing the family together. One way round this might be to spend some time asking all of the family members the same question in turn. This may appear to be a cumbersome process, but it conveys the value placed on everyone's opinion and can provide a greater depth of information compared with a series of questions to the most involved parent.

Another type of question that can be usefully employed in family meetings is to ask family members to answer from the perspective of another. For example, asking an adolescent girl to speculate on why her father gets so angry when she stays out overnight not only provides information for the professional but also for different members of the family. This technique, if used carefully, can also be used to include family members who are opting out of the conversation by asking the others to think about the situation from their perspective. It highlights a principle of families: that if something happens to one individual, it impacts on others.

CONCLUDING FAMILY MEETINGS

Taking into account the different views and perspectives of the family can be time consuming and it is advisable not to try to cover too much in one meeting. The varied agendas and expectations of the family as outlined earlier mean that they will take away different impressions from the interview. They may feel that someone else's view has been given a better hearing than their own. A useful technique is to put aside some time at the end of the meeting to ask each member of the family if there is something important that has not been raised. While there may not be sufficient time to explore any of these issues in any depth, they will have been raised and can be revisited at further meetings.

It is a considerable task to gather together all of the information from a family meeting especially if you are working alone. Checking your understanding of what has been said during the meeting by asking the family at the end of the meeting can be a good way to summarise and clarify any points of information. It also helps clarify whether younger members of the family have understood what has happened and what the plan is to deal with the issues.

Case study: Samuel

Samuel is eight years old and has been missing a lot of school recently due to illness. Accompanied by his mother he frequently consults his GP who can find nothing wrong with him. As a primary health worker you have arranged a meeting with Sam and his parents with the aim of devising some strategies to help him to get back into school on a more regular basis. The day before the scheduled meeting Sam's mother telephones to ask if they all need to attend.

How would you respond?

The meeting goes ahead and you start by asking about the problem. Sam's mother describes her worries and she becomes tearful. At the same time you notice that Sam is sinking lower and lower in his chair and his father is looking detached.

A mental health assessment

A standard mental health assessment plan is outlined below. Depending on the information already available, some parts may require greater inquiry than others. Some areas may need revisiting if new evidence comes to light or the problem identified does not resolve with appropriate intervention. Primary care staff are unlikely to undertake detailed or formal mental health assessments. The assessment is included here for primary care staff to be aware of what the assessment comprises so that they can adequately prepare young people and families they refer to CAMHS.

History taking

- **Presenting problem**

Need to establish the history of the presenting problem: onset, duration, severity, and associated factors, situations that improve or exacerbate the situation.

For whom is it a problem and what are associated issues?

What have the family and child already tried to make things better?

- **Family history**

Who is in the family?

Contact with absent parents.

Young people's perceptions of the family including their perceptions of any family behaviours, problems or breakdown.

Parents' own experiences of being parented.

Support within the family and extended family.

Roles and relationships within the family.

Communication within the family.

Issues of domestic violence.

Family history of mental health problems.

- **Personal history**

Prenatal, perinatal and postnatal history (i.e. details of the pregnancy and birth).

Development history – were milestones reached within expected time range?

School career, including how they separated from parents, settled into the school routine, relationships with peers and teachers and educational achievements.

Social interests and hobbies.

Social and peer relationships.

- **Past psychiatric and medical history**

When asking about previous episodes ask about what interventions were used and if these were successful. Ask about reasons for the interventions being useful or not. Record use of any prescribed or non-prescribed medication.

- **Substance use**

Include any contact with the police or legal services and medical and social consequences of use.

- **Contact with other agencies**

Such as social services, education, voluntary agencies and other health agencies.

- **Aspects of the young person before the onset of the problem**

Such as temperament; history of achievements. A useful question here can be to ask how the young person would use three wishes. This can help identify the young person's priorities.

Formal mental state examination

A formal mental state examination is an essential part of a specialist assessment, but any professional should be able to record the presentation accurately, although they may not have the training to interpret it. Details of observed behaviour are an essential part of the assessment.

A child psychiatrist should make the mental state examination. Avoid making pejorative or unnecessary personal comments about the young person. State what evidence you have to support your conclusions – record the behaviours rather than just your interpretation of them. The following should be noted:

- **General observations**

Appearance and behaviour.

How the young person engaged with the professional.

Levels of cooperation, concentration, anxiety and nervousness.

- **Speech**

Tone, rhythm, pace and volume.

Clarity, syntax and structure.

- **Mood**

Objective (observed by professional, including apparent general mood state and its range, depth and reactivity).

Subjective (young person's perceptions of their mood).

- **Disorders of perceptions**

Hallucinations – auditory (including whether there are any voices giving commands, or making derogatory or persecutory comments), visual, somatic (i.e. internal bodily sensations), tactile (skin), olfactory (smell) or gustatory (taste).

- **Disorder of thought form**

Speed of thought, linking of ideas.

- **Disorder of thought content**

Overvalued ideas, ideas of reference (i.e. that other things or people refer to them).

Delusions (fixed beliefs made on false premise that are not culturally contextual) – these may be grandiose, paranoid (persecutory), nihilistic, self-derogatory or religious. There may be delusions of passivity (believing that the mind or body is controlled in some way).

Obsessions (uncontrollable and intrusive thoughts, impulses or images that recur and cause significant distress and anxiety).

- **Cognition**

Orientation in time, place and person.

Memory and concentration.

Language and comprehension.

Visio-spatial skills.

Judgement and reasoning.

- **Safety of self and others**

It is *essential* that professionals at all levels ask young people about thoughts of harm to self or others, including suicidal and homicidal ideation. Asking about such thoughts does not make a young person more likely to act on them. Indeed, asking may do the opposite, as a professional raising the issue will reduce the young person's sense of isolation, and permit planning around how to manage the risk. Young people are often relieved at having been able to share what has been a considerable burden. There is greater risk in not asking than asking.

Psychometric assessment

Screening and other psychometric instruments can be useful in indicating the possibility of a disorder; however, they should not and cannot replace a thorough assessment.

Formulation

The mental health assessment is followed by a formulation, which integrates all the information, making sense of the problem or diagnosis, and highlighting relevant predisposing, precipitating and perpetuating factors in a way that enables a management plan to be devised. A good formulation sets out to answer the questions: *why this person?*, *why this presentation?* and *why now?*

Assessing young people with problem substance use

Young people access specialist services through front-line professionals in primary care settings, and these professionals are best placed to identify problems. Screening tools are available, such as the SACS (Christie *et al.* 2006). A professional concerned about a young person's substance use

---

RAFFT screening questionnaire to screen for substance use

(described by Liepman *et al.* 1998)

R   Do you ever take drugs to **R**elax, feel better about yourself or fit in?

A   Do you ever drink or take drugs while you are **A**lone?

F   Do any of your closest **F**riends drink or use drugs?

F   Does a close **F**amily member have a problem with alcohol or drugs?

T   Have you ever got into **T**rouble from drinking or taking drugs?

If the young person or his/her parents respond 'yes' to any of the above screening questions it may be useful to consider specialist services and also consider if the responses raise any child-protection concerns.

---

should be open to discussing the issue with the young person. There is strong evidence that this enables young people to access services. Initially, this assessment needs to clarify a young person's substance use so that accurate and up-to-date information and advice can be given if needed. A young person with problem substance use requires a comprehensive assessment by a professional who has the appropriate skills.

As well as identifying mental health needs, assessment should identify pattern and history of substance use, adverse consequences for the young person, risk factors to perpetuating use, beliefs held by the young person, and resources and strengths that can be called on to support the young person's aims in addressing the problem use.

Making a diagnosis

Unless they have the appropriate professional background and training, tier-one staff should refrain from making a diagnosis as families may find it difficult to relinquish the diagnosis even if specialist assessment proves otherwise. It is more helpful to discuss with the family the reasons for a referral to CAMHS.

References

Association of American Medical Colleges (1999) *Report III. Contemporary Issues in Medicine: Communication in Medicine.* Medical School Objectives Project. Washington, DC: Association of American Medical Colleges.

Christie, G., Marsh, R., Sheridan, J., Wheeler, A., Suaalii-Sauni, T., Black, S. and Butler, R. (2006) *The Substances and Choices Scale Manual.* Wellington: Alcohol Advisory Council. Available at www.sacsinfo.com/docs/SACSUserManualNoPrint.pdf, accessed on 18 July 2008.

Department of Health (2001) *Seeking Consent: Working With Children.* London: Department of Health. Available at www.doh.gov.uk/en/Publicationsandstatistics/Publications/PublicationsPolicyAndGuidance/DH_4007005, accessed on 18 July 2008.

Dogra, N. (2007) 'Cultural diversity issues.' In P. Vostanis (ed.) *Mental Health Interventions and Services for Vulnerable Children and Young People.* London: Jessica Kingsley Publishers.

Liepman, M.R., Keller, D.M., Botelho, R.J., Monroe, A.D. and Sloane, M.A. (1998) 'Understanding and preventing substance abuse by adolescents: A guide for primary care clinicians.' *Primary Care; Clinics in Office Practice 25*, 1, 137–162.

Pearce, J. (1994) 'Consent to treatment during childhood. The assessment of competence and avoidance of conflict.' *British Journal of Psychiatry 165*, 713–716.

Further reading

British Medical Association (2001) *Consent, Rights and Choices in Health Care for Children and Young People.* London: BMJ Books.

Burnham, J. (1996) *Family Therapy: First Steps Towards a Systematic Approach.* London: Routledge.

Graham, P. (1993) *Child Psychiatry: A Developmental Approach* (2nd edition). New York: Oxford University Press.

Hobday, A. and Ollier, K. (1998) *Creative Therapy: Activities with Children and Adolescents.* Leicester: BPS Books.

Hobday, A. and Ollier, K. (1999) *Creative Therapy 2: Working with Parents.* Leicester: BPS Books.

Kendall, R.E. (1998) 'Diagnosis and classification.' In R.E. Kendall and A.K. Zeally (eds) *Companion to Psychiatric Studies* (4th edition). Edinburgh: Churchill Livingstone.

Maguire, G.P. (1998) 'The psychiatric interviews.' In R.E. Kendall and A.K. Zeally (eds) *Companion to Psychiatric Studies* (4th edition). Edinburgh: Churchill Livingstone.

McCrum, S. and Hughes, L. (1998) *Interviewing Children* (2nd edition). London: Save the Children.

Rutter, M., Taylor, E. and Hersov, L. (1994) *Child and Adolescent Psychiatry: Modern Approaches* (3rd edition). Oxford: Blackwell Scientific.

Swadi, H. (2000) 'Substance misuse in adolescents.' *Advances in Psychiatric Treatment 6,* 201–210.

Worden, M. (1998) *Family Therapy Basics.* Pacific Grove, CA: Brooks/Cole.

PART 2

Child and Family Development

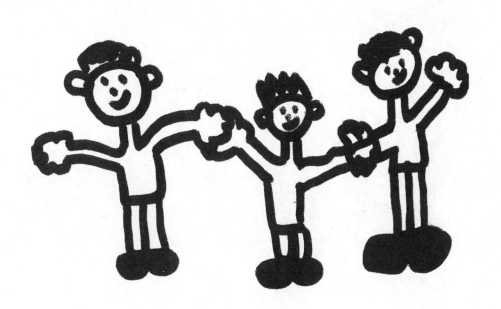

CHAPTER 4

Child and Adolescent Development

Psychological development in childhood

An understanding of psychological development underpins concepts in mental health throughout the lifespan as well as being crucial to understanding developmental delay. Psychological development begins at birth, or even before, and continues through to old age. As with physical development, there are periods of particularly rapid development in childhood and adolescence, which is what will be focused on in this section. However, it should be remembered that whilst physical development stops after adolescence, psychological development continues throughout the lifespan. Physical and psychological development are closely related throughout – from the coordination of motor and perceptual function in early childhood with increased exploration of the world and the child's developing identity in relation to that, to the changes at puberty and the physical and psychological sequelae of that. The relationship between physical development and psychological development should be borne in mind throughout, although the former is not described here. Once we have discussed development, we will also briefly review developmental delay as these children have an increased likelihood of developing mental health problems.

Children's developing concept that they and other people have mental states is known as 'theory of mind' and is described first as it is relevant to all aspects of psychological development. Cognitive, emotional, social and moral development will then be considered in turn. Table 4.1 summarises the theories of development described in this section.

Table 4.1 Comparison of developmental theories in childhood

AGE	ERIKSEN	PIAGET	VYGOTSKY	THEORY OF MIND	KOHLBERG
0 – 1	Trust vs. mistrust	Sensori-motor	Pre-intellectual speech		Punishment and reward orientations
1 – 2	Autonomy vs. shame and doubt				
2 – 3		Preoperational	Practical intelligence	Capable of deception	
3 – 4	Initiative vs. guilt			Distinguish thoughts/objects/perceptions/knowledge	
4 – 5			Use of external symbols	Pass false belief tests: people hold different beliefs	
5 – 6	Industry vs. inferiority				
6 – 7				Distinguish fantasy/reality more reliably	
7 – 8		Concrete operational	Internal dialogue	Understand different interpretations. Link thoughts	Good child and authority orientations
8 – 9				Understand inference	
9 – 10					
10 – 11				Understand basic nature of other cognitive processes	
11 – 12	Identity vs. confusion	Formal operational			
12 – 13					Social contact and ethical principle orientations
13 – 14					
14+				Distinguish problem solving/hypothesis testing	

Ages given throughout this chapter serve as indicators of when skills develop but they should not be taken as fixed as children develop at different rates.

Theory of mind

'Theory of mind' is the understanding that oneself and others have mental states, that is recognising that other people also have thoughts and feelings, and eliciting clues to these from their social behaviour.

- From the age of two or three years a child begins to learn that it is possible to deceive others – cognitive deception (misrepresenting or hiding information).

- By the age of four years a child recognises that thoughts about an object are distinct from the object itself and that thoughts, perceptions and knowledge are different from each other. Similarly, the differentiation of experienced and expressed emotion emerges at the same age. It is not until a year later that they begin to understand that others may hold different beliefs (i.e. pass 'false belief tasks'). Preschool children rarely acknowledge their own or others' thinking, even when given cues to this. Children may be unable to distinguish fantasy from reality until beyond 6 years.

- It is not until the age of seven or eight years that children recognise that one thought may trigger another ('stream of consciousness'), that this is only partly controllable, and that events/places/memories may trigger thoughts ('cognitive cueing'). Around this age children recognise that different interpretations may be placed on the same event or phrase (e.g. they begin to understand more sophisticated jokes involving puns).

- By the age of eight years children have developed a basic understanding of inference – that another thought or desire may lie behind a statement or action (e.g. looking longingly at a box of chocolates when they want to eat one, or saying, 'That looks like a fun toy', meaning they want to play with the toy).

- It is not until after ten years of age that children develop an understanding of the basic nature of other cognitive processes (such as different types of memory, reasoning, attention and comprehension). The ability to develop between different cognitive processes continues through adolescence and into adulthood.

Cognitive development

Cognitions may be simply described as 'mental processes'. These include understanding, believing, calculating, knowing, creating, reasoning, generating ideas, inferring, conceptualising, fantasising and dreaming, as well as coordinating motor function and perception. Three theories on cognitive development have greatly influenced this area: Piagetian theory, information processing and Vygotskian theory.

PIAGETIAN THEORY

Piaget (1950) described four phases of development that are universal, and that develop at much the same rate irrespective of environmental influences. His theory influenced educational practice internationally. The phases result from the interaction between the maturation of the central nervous system, physical experience, social interaction, and a psychological homeostatic mechanism. The last allows equilibration, which is the incorporation of new experiences into previously held concepts. Piaget suggested that cognitive development depends on several steps:

1. *assimilation* – relating new information to previous understanding

2. *accommodation* – changing the prior understanding as a result of new information

3. *adaptation* – responding to this in new situations.

The four phases of development from birth to early adolescence described by Piaget require increasingly conceptual skills, and not everyone reaches the same potential within each phase. They are based on observations and experiments he conducted, and have since been tested in other studies.

- **Phase 1: Sensori-motor (birth–2 years)**

The child begins to associate and integrate perceptions and motor actions, for example movement of the arm occurs with visual stimuli and a sense of limb position (proprioception), which suggest to the child that this arm is part of his or her body and can be controlled by him or her. They understand that objects still exist, even when they can no longer see them. The development of such concepts is assisted across cultures by games such as 'peek-a-boo'.

- **Phase 2: Preoperational (2–7 years)**

From late toddlerhood through to the early preschool years children enter this phase, in which they can make mental representations of objects and imagine the actions associated with them. Their view of the world is egocentric, meaning they see themselves as having a greater influence on events than they have in reality, and vice versa.

- **Phase 3: Concrete operational (7–11 years)**

In the next phase from middle to late childhood, thoughts are logical and coordinated. The child remains 'concrete' in his or her thinking, meaning that he or she is limited to tangible and fixed concepts. The development of concepts such as 'the preservation of volume' can be demonstrated at this age; for example, a child who has developed this will recognise that water poured from a tall thin jug into a short wide jug remains the same in volume. A younger child witnessing the same demonstration would state that there is more water in the tall thin glass because the level is higher.

- **Phase 4: Formal operational (11 years and up)**

From about 11 years old, children enter the final phase, in which they are able to think in abstract terms. In this phase, children can begin to apply concepts that are beyond their direct experience, make prepositional statements that follow a logical argument and test out their own hypotheses, such as about the physical properties of objects.

INFORMATION PROCESSING

Information processing is a cognitive function whereby information is recognised, coded, stored, and retrieved. Very young children use very basic processes, with the development of deliberate strategic approaches in later childhood. The mind functions as a set of parallel 'units' working contemporaneously, with each unit representing a small item of information. Each unit may represent, for instance, one characteristic of a familiar object (e.g. texture of a blanket). Several units relating to one object may be located in different parts of the brain. These units of information may relate directly to each other without the need for a centralised control. Thus, the mind constantly re-evaluates and collates information.

VYGOTSKIAN THEORY

Vygotsky (1978) described the dependence of cognitive development (including thinking, memory and attention) upon external factors, such as the social environment, which includes the context of guiding adults who 'scaffold' the child's development. This approach recognises the close links between cognitive, social and language development. Cognitive development depends on the child making active use of social interactions and internalising these. Thus, 'internal' (cognitive) development depends on 'external' (social) interaction, not the other way round – in contrast with the ideas of Piaget and information processing theory. Four phases are identified:

1.   Infants and toddlers (up to two years) use vocal activity as a means of social contact and emotional expression: this is known as 'pre-intellectual speech' and 'preverbal thought'.

2.   The second phase is the development of 'practical intelligence' with loose links between use of language and problem solving.

3.   Later, children start to use symbols external to themselves to assist internal problem solving, for example talking oneself through problems, finger counting.

4.   These are finally internalised, as language is then used in internal dialogue to develop thought and reflect (though external tools are still used for difficult problems).

Emotional development

The preschool years are a period of particularly rapid development, as for many aspects of psychological development. Emotional development is a complex area, which is best described by detailing the tasks that a child needs to accomplish.

The tasks of emotional development include:

- recognising the significance of emotions and differentiating between emotion states (i.e. combination of feelings, associated behaviours and level of arousal) in self and others

- learning to contain emotions and the socio-culturally appropriate and acceptable expression of emotions (the regulation of emotions); and, as a result, distinguishing between emotions experienced and emotions expressed, both in self and in others

- understanding the impact of emotions on behaviour and relationships (the regulatory capacity of emotions).

DEVELOPMENT OF DIFFERENTIATION OF EMOTIONS
Differentiating between emotions

- has a biological significance in terms of survival or learning
- proceeds from birth (and possibly before)
- is difficult to assess in preverbal ages
- is more reliably demonstrated for 'complex' emotions in later childhood.

The ages at which a reliable understanding of each emotion is achieved are given in Table 4.2.

THE EXPRESSION, CONCEALMENT AND SHARING OF EMOTION
Learning to contain and appropriately express emotion is learnt from parents and peers both by direct intervention (e.g. parental management of tantrums) and vicariously (e.g. observation of adults' and peers' emotional responses to a situation). Learning to regulate emotions in this way is a lifelong process, but is of paramount importance throughout childhood and adolescence.

At a preschool age the development of learning when and how to hide feelings probably occurs simultaneously with an understanding that others can also do this. This is partly dependent on the development of theory of mind, and is akin to the understanding of cognitive deception. As well as being regulated, emotions are regulatory. They may influence

Table 4.2 Emotions consistently identified by children with age
(after work by Harris *et al.* 1987)

Emotion	Age from which each emotion is included (years)
Happy	5+
Sad	
Afraid	
Angry	
Shy	
Proud	
Worried	7+
Grateful	
Excited	
Surprised	
Jealous	
Guilty	
Disappointed	10+
Curious	
Relieved	
Disgusted	
Ashamed	14+
Shocked	
Embarrassed	
Depressed	

interpretation of events, potential responses to events or situations, and behaviour of the individual and others. Notable steps in emotional development are:

- *from birth to 18 months* – emotional state can be determined by behavioural responses (e.g. parents can distinguish specific cries and vocalisations, which they understand to convey different needs)

- *from 18 to 24 months* – expression of first words describing emotions

- *at around 2 years* – increase in the use of pretend play to express feelings and frequent expression of anger or frustration through tantrums

- *by 3 years* – competence at talking with parents, siblings, and peers about feelings (this varies with parents' use of words to describe emotions); frequent use of play or humour, gesture and facial expression to express emotion.

The ability to share emotions (i.e. the mutual expression and registration of feelings) in early childhood facilitates the resolution of difficult emotions, which leads to enhanced understanding and regulation of emotions, which leads to ability to provide constructive responses to conflict, and predicts increased cooperation in later childhood and possibly adulthood.

The ability to share emotions with peers about third parties (e.g. disgust), is apparent by the age of five years and predicts acceptance by friends and peers, which in turn predicts the self-regulation of 'difficult' emotions such as anger, anxiety and fear. This interaction between social and emotional development continues throughout childhood. By the age of ten years there is increased sharing between friends of socially undesirable feelings in a socially acceptable manner. As children develop they increasingly share emotional experiences and memories with a same-gender friend (or small group of friends), deriving relief from being 'understood' and enhancing the friendship. A child is more likely than an adult to understand the emotional expression of a peer of the same stage of development, which may explain the potency of therapeutic groups.

Social development

Social development is interdependent with other aspects of development. There are two broad ways of describing social development. One is by plotting the tasks of social development throughout the lifespan, which Eriksen (1965) first described. The other is by examining the details of social interaction (see 'Social skills' below), and how this influences peer relationships. The nature of attachment influences social development, the relationships that young people have with peers and adults, and how this subsequently develops in adult life. Attachment and attachment disorders are described in Chapters 6 and 8.

ERIKSEN'S 'EIGHT STAGES OF MAN'

Eriksen (1965) described the 'Eight Stages of Man', a model for socio-emotional development in humans. Longitudinal cohort studies of up to 80 years have demonstrated the validity of these concepts in 'Western society'. Moving on to each stage is not dependent on complete resolution of tasks and conflicts in previous stages. The stages relevant to childhood are:

1. **Basic trust vs. mistrust (first year of life)**

    The child will develop trust in the world if his/her needs are predictably met. Otherwise, the child may develop a perception of the world as a hostile and unpredictable place. Gross deprivation at this stage may lead to emotional detachment in childhood and throughout life, with difficulties forming deep and lasting relationships in adulthood.

2. **Autonomy vs. shame and doubt (1–3 years)**

    The child acquires confidence in his/her own ability as opposed to self-doubt. The child begins to recognise his/her own will, and ability to be independent; and may feel guilt if he/she does not conform to expected behaviours. This stage is about learning to balance one's own wishes against those of others. Failing to exert oneself may lead to reduced confidence and initiative, but failure to take into account others' wishes may make it difficult to integrate into society fully.

3. **Initiative vs. guilt (3–5 years)**

   The child acquires more social skills and assumes greater responsibility for self. A sense of time begins to develop. The child builds on the tasks accomplished in the previous stage. Successful resolution at this stage results in a confident and outgoing child. Others may develop fears or problems with nightmares as they struggle to resolve the conflict.

4. **Industry vs. inferiority (5–11 years)**

   The challenge here is to achieve and overcome feelings of failure. The child will be industrious in schoolwork, sport and social relationships. If these are not achieved the child may feel a sense of failure and inferiority. He/she may also become isolated from the peer group.

5. **Identity vs. confusion (11+ years)**

   In this stage the child acquires a firm sense of who he/she is (separate from the family), what he/she wants from life and where he/she is going. This is further discussed in adolescent development.

The three remaining stages for completeness are: intimacy vs. isolation (young adulthood), generativity vs. stagnation (middle adulthood), and integrity vs. despair (old age).

SOCIAL SKILLS

Essential social skills include eye contact, turn taking, listening, interaction in play, learning appropriate behaviour and physical contact. These in turn influence popularity, peer relationships and friendships. To respond to another child's social behaviour, a child needs to follow six steps:

1. encode that behaviour

2. interpret it

3. search for appropriate responses

4. evaluate and select a response

5. enact the response

6. monitor outcome.

This is similar to the steps described in information processing in cognitive development. The successful development of peer relationships is partly dependent on these skills.

PEER RELATIONSHIPS AND PLAY

Peer relationships vary in quality and size, and their nature shows development throughout childhood. Both popularity and friendships depend upon behavioural and emotional interactions, which in childhood are exercised through play.

Children are initially closely monitored and moderated by parents or other adults. Infants and toddlers will hold on to an attachment figure while looking at (i.e. being interested in) peers. Adults 'scaffold' early infant–infant interaction. From two to four years, skills increase with age, largely through play. Initially mainly rough-and-tumble, this develops into pretend role-play (socio-dramatic play). Play develops from toddlerhood to school age in four identifiable stages:

1. solitary play (child plays by self)
2. parallel play (child plays alongside others, may mimic, etc.)
3. associative play (child plays with others, but without organised structure)
4. cooperative play (child plays with others with routine, acceptance of rules, and 'productively').

Peer group size increases with age, earlier in girls than boys. The quality of interactions changes throughout childhood with the development of identifiable groups of friends.

POPULARITY

Popularity is relatively stable over time and can be measured by ascertaining the perceptions children have of each other in their peer groups. Five groups can be distinguished on this basis and are shown in Figure 4.1.

Popularity is influenced by characteristics of both the group as a whole, and the individual child. These include physical attractiveness, obesity, handicap and temperament. Social withdrawal may have an inter-active causal association with dislike of a child by the peer group.

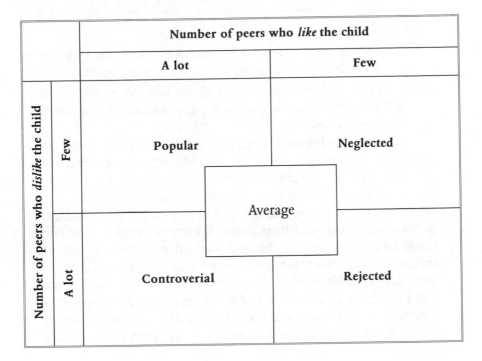

Figure 4.1 Peer popularity

The use of the six steps of social skills differs between the five groups. For instance, popular children follow through the six steps. Neglected children encode and interpret, but may go no further. Rejected children 'crash in' at stage 5, often with an inappropriate response of which peers are intolerant. Controversial children often follow through, but are erratic in their responses. They are often bullies or bully-victims.

FRIENDSHIPS

Friendships develop from toddlerhood. Their development has three identifiable stages:

1. reward–cost basis (usually up to 8 years) – for example, with shared activities, live near by

2. normative (entered at 9–10 years) with shared values, rules and sanctions

3. empathic (entered at 11–12 years) with increased understanding between friends, self-disclosure and shared interests.

Case study: Sunil

Sunil is an eight-year-old child who lives with his parents. The extended family is very close, with most family members living nearby. Sunil developed a very close relationship with his paternal grandparents, visiting them daily. When he was seven years old, both grandparents died in a road accident.

Sunil's parents found this extremely difficult to cope with, and his mother in particular found it very difficult to talk about her in-laws, or to have any photographs or memories of them around the house. Sunil attended the cremation and found it confusing. It became very clear to him that every time he brought up the subject of his grandparents and their death, his mother either burst into tears, became angry, or changed the subject. Therefore Sunil stopped talking about them, because he thought this would be the most helpful to his mother. At school, teachers noted that he was more isolated and distant, and that the quality of his schoolwork deteriorated. This continued for a number of weeks, but whenever his teacher asked him whether there was any problem, he would deny it.

Eventually, Sunil's parents took him to see his GP because he was becoming increasingly irritable and aggressive towards them. When seen on his own, Sunil told the GP that he was very sad that his grand-parents were not alive, and he wondered whether he had been responsible for their death. A referral was made to the local child and family psychiatric service and the whole family was seen. It became clear that Sunil's parents had felt unable to help Sunil with his grief because of the difficulty that they were having. Sunil's parents agreed to a referral to Cruse (a bereavement counselling agency) for bereavement counselling in their own right, and Sunil was seen individually on six occasions every two weeks. During that time Sunil was able to clarify a number of his misperceptions and explore his own grief. This led to a resolution of many of his symptoms of irritability, poor concentration and physical aggression. Through their attendance at Cruse, Sunil's parents them-selves also managed to move on through this grieving process.

What concerns did Sunil have, and what are the related developmental issues?

What is the role of a specialist CAMHS in a presentation like this?

Friendships from early childhood predict the quality of friendships in later childhood and adulthood. Low peer acceptance also predicts early school drop out and, more controversially, higher rates of juvenile and adult crime. Friendships from middle childhood onwards are mostly formed on a mutually voluntary basis. Children expect, and benefit, differentially from friendships. Companionship is a common characteristic, with increased provision of emotional support and intimacy with increased age.

Moral development

Relatively less has been written on moral development. Most work in this area is based on Kohlberg's model.

KOHLBERG'S MODEL

Kohlberg (1973) applied Piaget's theories to develop a framework for moral development. This theory more accurately describes the development of moral reasoning rather than moral behaviour. Although this theory is based on cognitive development, moral development is very closely interwoven with social development. Kohlberg described three levels of moral development:

- **Level I Pre-conventional morality**

Stage 1: punishment orientation (child obeys rules to avoid punishment)

Stage 2: reward orientation (child conforms to expectations to have rewards)

- **Level II Conventional morality**

Stage 3: good child orientation (child conforms to avoid disapproval of others)

Stage 4: authority orientation (upholds laws and rules to avoid censure of authorities)

- **Level III Post-conventional morality**

Stage 5: social contact orientation (actions guided by principles commonly agreed on as essential to public welfare; principles upheld to retain respect of peers)

Stage 6: ethical principle orientation (actions guided by self-chosen ethical principles that usually value justice, dignity and equality; principles are upheld to retain self-respect).

It is important to distinguish between the development of moral concepts and changes in behaviour. The two are usually interdependent, but both should be assessed.

Adolescent development

Adolescence is loosely defined as a period of transition from puberty (around 11 years of age) to late teens or early twenties. It is, however, culturally and historically variable. In Western societies, adolescence is generally seen as a time of transition from childhood to adulthood. There may be transitions that all young people experience (such as leaving school) or some that only happen to some individuals (such as experiencing parental divorce). There may be internal changes (such as biological changes of puberty) or external ones (such as expectations of society). The changes may be normative (that is expected to occur at a particular age physiologically or as prescribed culturally) or idiosyncratic (person specific, such as illness). The transitions may be on time or off time and unexpected or expected. Generally, on time and expected changes are less disruptive than off time and unexpected transitions. There is consistent evidence that most young people manage the transition of adolescence without undue stress. Some of the behaviours of adolescence may be focused on because of the discomfort they generate in adults. Media representation of adolescents can also distort the realities.

In Western societies the tasks of adolescence can be defined as follows:

1. increasing educational demands and establishing adult vocational goals and thinking about how to achieve them (this may also mean preparing for financial independence and a career)

2. adjustment to being a sexually mature adult (this includes developing sexual identity, sexual orientation and sexuality)

3. developing peer relationships (sexual and non-sexual)

4. developing a personal sense of identity

5. acquiring a personal set of values and ethical system, a personal ideology

6. increasing responsibility for one's own behaviour, which usually means desiring and achieving socially responsible behaviour

7. achieving independence from parents and other adults (emotional, psychological, financial and otherwise)

8. preparing for one's own marriage and family (can be widely interpreted and still applies to most young people).

Tasks are culturally specific to an extent and may present conflict to some individuals, for example developing a sense of one's own sexuality and there being a societal expectation that one should be heterosexual.

Biological change is necessary for some of the above tasks to be completed (e.g. 1, 2, 7 and 8). Some degree of psychological maturity is needed for all tasks. External conditions may strongly impact on tasks 1, 5, 7 and 8 (economic conditions may dictate employment, and although an individual may be ready to separate from their parents, their personal finances may make that impossible). Socio-cultural forces are reflected in all the tasks as each involves social expectations and definitions.

In early adolescence there is rapid physical and intellectual growth. In middle adolescence there is increasing self-reliance, more intimate friendships and dating may begin. By late adolescence a clear consistent sense of self has usually developed with ideas on roles and value systems as well as personal life goals. There are phases of adolescent maturity and these anticipate that between 10 and 13 years most young people are compliant with expectations of them. Rebellion usually occurs between 14 and 17 years. Between 17 and 21 years most young people mature and outgrow their need to rebel. Whether adolescents successfully complete the tasks expected of them will also to some extent depend on the way their parents

---

Case study: Alison

Alison is 15 years old and has been complaining of a loss of interest in her schoolwork. She is questioning the point of being at school and feels it has no relevance to her now or for the future. You have known Alison for some time and this is quite a change from how you have seen her.

What would you do?

What might Alison's lack of interest be related to?

After talking to Alison, you think she is confused about her sexuality. What would you do next?

---

respond to the task. Parents may struggle with balancing the task of providing autonomy for the young person while still retaining a degree of control. Young people may also challenge the long-held value systems of their parents, thus leading to conflict. Interestingly, early puberty presents greater problems for girls than boys, and late puberty appears to present more difficulties for boys than girls.

Developmental delay

Developmental disorders can be classified into two groups, which will be outlined in turn:

- general developmental delay
- specific developmental disorders.

General developmental delay

CHARACTERISTICS AND PRESENTATION

Terminology for this changes frequently in an attempt to avoid stigmatisation. It is now commonly known in the UK as *learning disability* (LD) and more recently as *developmental disability*, but is also referred to as mental handicap, or mental retardation. It is characterised by:

- global delay/slowing/hindered development (i.e. affecting all areas of physical, intellectual and psychological development)
- preservation of the sequence of development.

General developmental delay can present at different ages:

- routine antenatal screening for Down syndrome, congenital abnormalities
- specific (at risk) antenatal screening of metabolic and genetic disorders
- at birth – physical characteristics of disorders commonly associated with LD (such as Down syndrome)
- preschool – delay in expected milestones
- school-age – delayed speech/social development; poor scholastic achievement.

ASSESSMENT AND DIAGNOSIS

The assessment is more than simply a measure of intelligence and should take into account the child's ability to function physically, socially, in activities of daily living and self-care, such as washing and dressing, as well as academically. Further medical investigation of the known causes of developmental delay (see below) should be made.

Diagnosis requires the following:

1. Onset before age 18 years.

2. A significant reduced level of intellectual functioning. A commonly accepted measure of intelligence is IQ (intelligence quotient) although there are concerns about its application and validity in different populations (Victor 2000). Table 4.3 shows the categories of intellectual functioning. However, assessment of severity should also take account of general adaptive functioning, without over-reliance on a single measure of function such as IQ.

3. Diminished ability to adapt to daily demands in areas such as self-care, communication, social competence, etc.

A comprehensive assessment of functioning as a minimum requires physical and mental state examinations, information from parents and teachers, and observation in various environments. There may be additional need for more detailed testing of specific areas of function. This assessment must take account of cultural expectations and expected functioning for age. Assessment can be assisted by standardised informant-report inventories gathering information from parents or others who know the child well (such as the Vineland Adaptive Behaviour Scale [Sparrow, Balla and Cicchetti 1984]).

Table 4.3 IQ and severity of learning disability

IQ	Severity of learning disability
50–69	Mild
35–49	Moderate
20–34	Severe
<20	Profound

CAUSES OF LEARNING DISABILITY

There are two broad groups: inherited and acquired. These can be broken down further:

Inherited

- Chromosomal disorders, chromosomal abnormalities (chromosomes are large packages of genetic material). Any syndrome characterised by malformation or malfunction in any of the body's systems may be caused by an abnormality in the number or structure of the chromosomes, for example Down syndrome (there is an extra chromosome) and fragile X syndrome (the structure of the X chromosome is altered).

- Genetic, causing chemical imbalances, such as phenylketonuria.

- Physical abnormalities, such as hydrocephalus and neurofibromatosis.

Acquired

- Infection, such as rubella and encephalitis.

- Trauma, such as radiation, birth asphyxia, accidental or non-accidental injury.

- Poisoning, such as lead intoxication.

- Malnutrition.

- Environmental factors, such as poverty, poor housing, unstable family or understimulation.

More than one factor may mediate learning disability. Psychological and environmental factors may account for variation in IQ of as much as 20

Case study: Julie

Julie is a seven-year-old girl who was brought to the attention of the educational welfare officer (EWO) as her school attendance had gradually fallen to less than 25 per cent. The EWO learnt that Julie frequently attended her GP with non-specific 'ailments', often complaining that she could not do her schoolwork because of these. Her mother was anxious, often kept Julie off school because of this, and believed her difficulties were due to 'dyslexia', 'vitamin deficiency', and a list of some very rare and unusual disorders. Julie's school reported that she was markedly behind in her schoolwork and had not made friends. She could not yet write her name or simple words, had poor pencil skills and could barely read books for preschool children. On further enquiry, Julie's mother reluctantly admitted that she still needed to dress Julie and assist her using cutlery.

Who should next assess Julie?

What is the likely diagnosis?

Why do you think Julie's mother sought so many explanations for her difficulties?

Why do you think Julie had so many non-specific physical ailments?

What interventions would you recommend?

points. Studies of institutionalised young people suggest that providing more stimulating home and school environments can significantly increase IQ (Capron and Duyme 1989; Dumaret 1985; Garber 1988; Provence and Naylor 1983; Ramey, Campbell and Finkelstein 1984).

Specific Developmental Disorders

These include specific disorders of:

- *Speech and language* – if there are any concerns about articulation, expression or understanding of speech and language, a speech therapy assessment is required.

- *Reading, writing, spelling or arithmetic skills* – difficulties arise in establishing these as there are many confounding factors, such as an understimulating environment.

- *Motor function (physical movement)* – developmental disorders of motor function usually present with clumsiness, and there may be impairment of hand–eye coordination.

- *A combination of the above* – these all have an onset in the early stages of development, are commonly present early and are more common in boys. The specific delay should not be accounted for by a global developmental delay or pervasive developmental disorder (PDD). It is important to exclude medical causes, such as neurological and hearing abnormalities.

Strategies for use with developmental delay

Specific interventions in all types of developmental delay are largely aimed at maximising the young person's potential and supporting the family. Treatable causes of the delay should be identified. However, the majority of developmental delays are of unknown aetiology, and many known causes are untreatable.

Intervention to meet the young person's educational and social needs may include the provision of special education. In late adolescence and early adulthood, interventions may continue to focus on daily living skills with the provision of day care and sheltered housing. Issues of sex, sexuality and sexual orientation also need to be addressed.

Physical and mental health issues, including emotional and behavioural problems have a markedly higher prevalence in young people with a developmental delay. These often need specialist intervention, particularly for multiple and complex problems.

Behaviour therapy is commonly used to encourage the development of skills needed for self-reliance and to discourage behaviours such as self-injury and stereotopies (intentional but pointless movements carried out in a repetitive manner). It is particularly important when working with young people with learning disabilities to follow the ethical guidelines outlined in the section on behaviour management in Chapter 13. Consent should be sought from parents who should be fully involved in planning and implementation.

Young people with learning disabilities frequently use their behaviour to communicate. A good understanding of the function of the behaviour (in terms of what the young person gains or avoids) is essential to the planning of an intervention.

Family issues in delayed development

The interaction between the young person and their family (which may include unrelated peers and others) is important, with particular reference to family development, culture and individual temperament. Families with a child with a learning disability may have difficulty accomplishing the tasks in one or more stages of family development (outlined in Chapter 5). This may be as a result of an interruption to the usual pattern of parent–child interactions due to one or more of the following factors:

Factors in the young person:

- reduced readiness to participate in social interaction
- impaired perceptual abilities
- impaired motor function
- impairment of general arousal
- abnormal expression of features of attachment in the first year of life.

Factors in the parents

- parenting function impaired by guilt/depression/anxiety/grieving resulting in over-/under-involvement
- interruption of usual patterns of engagement from infancy, due either to parental failure to respond to the infant's socio-emotional needs because of lack of cues, or parental observation that their attempts fail to elicit the expected response in the infant.

These are important features to assess and may require specific intervention.

The role of temperament in delayed development

The categories and features of the temperaments of infants are outlined in more detail in Chapter 9. 'Difficult temperament' predisposes infants to behavioural and conduct problems. 'Slow-to-warm-up' temperament predisposes infants to emotional problems. An important mediating factor in this is the family's response to these features.

A cycle of increased negative emotional response, or of increased emotional distance between the child and other family members may perpetuate or exacerbate problem behaviours. The professional needs to understand the interactive nature of this cycle, elicit a clear history of family relationships and make interventions that reduce the problem behaviour and increase positive and appropriate behaviours. Parental stress and poor coping strategies may also need to be explored and support systems strengthened in order to allow the family to make the positive changes. The young person and their family may be aided by the provision of day services and activities or residential respite care

References

Capron, C. and Duyme, M. (1989) 'Assessment of effects of socio-economic status on IQ in a full cross-fostering study.' *Nature 340*, 552–554.

Dumaret, A. (1985) 'IQ, scholastic performance and behaviour of siblings raised in contrasting environments.' *Journal of Child Psychology and Psychiatry 26*, 553–580.

Eriksen, E. (1965) *Childhood and Society*. Harmondsworth: Penguin.

Garber, H.L. (1988) *The Milwaukee Project: Preventing Mental Retardation in Children at Risk*. Washington, DC: American Association of Mental Retardation.

Harris, P.L., Olthof, T., Meerum-Terwogt, M. and Hardman, C.E. (1987) 'Children's knowledge of the situations that provoke emotion.' *International Journal of Behavioural Development 10*, 319–343.

Kohlberg, L. (1973) *Collected Papers on Moral Development and Moral Education*. Cambridge, MA: Harvard University Press.

Piaget, J. (1950) *The Psychology of Intelligence*. London: Routledge and Kegan Paul.

Provence, S. and Naylor, A. (1983) *Working with Disadvantaged Parents and Children: Scientific Issues and Practice*. New Haven, CT: Yale University Press.

Ramey, C., Campbell, F. and Finkelstein, N. (1984). 'Course and structure of intellectual development in children at high risk for developmental retardation.' In P. Brooks, R. Sperber and C. McCauley (eds) *Learning and Cognition in the Mentally Retarded*. Hillsdale, NJ: Erlbaum.

Sparrow, S., Balla, D. and Cicchetti, D. (1984) *Vineland Adaptive Behaviour Scale*. Circle Pines, MN: American Guidance Service.

Victor, N. (2000) *Cross-cultural Neuropsychological Assessment: Theory and Practice*. Mahwah, NJ: Erlbaum.

Vygotsky, L.S. (1978) *Mind in Society: The Development of Higher Psychological Processes*. Cambridge, MA: Harvard University Press.

Further reading

Demetriou, A., Doise, W. and van Lieshout, C. (1998) *Life-span Developmental Psychology*. Chichester and New York: Wiley.

Gordon, J. and Grant, G. (eds) (1997) *How We Feel: An Insight into the Emotional World of Teenagers*. London: Jessica Kingsley Publishers.

Heaven, P.C.L. (1996) *Adolescent Health: The Role of Individual Differences*. London: Routledge.

Henderson, A. and Champlin, S. with Evashwick, W. (eds) (1998) *Promoting Teen Health: Linking Schools, Health Organizations and Community*. Thousand Oaks, CA: Sage.

Hinde, R.A. and Stevenson-Hinde, J. (1988) *Relationships within Families: Mutual Influences*. Oxford: Oxford Science Publications.

Kimmel, D.C. and Weiner, I.B. (1994) *Adolescence: A Developmental Transition* (2nd edition). New York: Wiley.

Mills, R. and Duck, S. (2000) *The Developmental Psychology of Personal Relationships*. Chichester and New York: Wiley.

CHAPTER 5

Family Development

Defining the family

Traditionally families have had at their heart a biological connection, but membership extends far beyond this. Indeed, it is impossible to define the extent of the family, as this is personally, legally and culturally determined. For example, some cultures may regard members of the extended family such as grandparents as an important influence in their day-to-day life, while other cultures would regard this as unhelpful and intrusive. There are many routes into a family such as birth, adoption, fostering, sexual relationships, and marriage. Generally speaking it is much easier to become a part of a family than it is to stop being part of one. Whatever value an individual places on their membership of a family, they can never completely leave it except through death.

In Western societies views on what is meant by family have been radically reshaped over the past few decades. In the UK there has been a dramatic increase in families headed by one parent. In the US stepfamilies now outnumber families made up of children living with both biological parents. In the UK there were nearly 150,000 divorces in 2006 and 53% of these couples had at least one child under 16 (Office for National Statistics 2005). This figure is an underestimate of this experience, as it does not take into account children of unmarried parents.

In many countries legal definitions of what constitutes a family still reflect a view that it should have as its basis a heterosexual married couple, as the rights and responsibilities of unmarried fathers and same-gender parenting couples are severely curtailed.

The increasing diversity of the ways people choose to live together, as seen in single parent families, same-gender couples, stepfamilies, and couples choosing not to marry, is gaining acceptance to varying degrees. The way that people live their lives is challenging the view of what is 'normal'. Nevertheless many families bear some resemblance to the 'traditional nuclear family' or are influenced by the idea in some way as this powerful image shapes expectations of family life.

Personal definitions of the family are not static, as we all need to make sense of our changing circumstances. As well as the common experience of joining a new family via a relationship there is also evidence from longitudinal studies of kinship networks that our views on family fluctuate depending on our differing needs throughout our lifetime.

For the purpose of working with children in a mental health context, a pragmatic definition of family would encompass all those involved in meeting the child's immediate emotional and developmental needs, which is a definition based on function rather than structure. This would usually include the household but can often extend to parents living elsewhere and, being mindful of issues of confidentiality, grandparents, close family friends, and child minders. Levin and Trost (1992) proposed a definition of family as two or more people who define themselves as family. In practice, families usually have little difficulty in defining themselves, but difficulties arise when the professional working with them does not share the family's views on membership because of their own cultural and personal expectations.

Family lifecycle

Much has been written on the development of the individual, and, whilst there are fewer theories on family development, the notion of a cyclical progression through an individual's life has wide acceptance across cultures and a similar model adapted to describe family life has proven to be a useful perspective on how families live their lives. Carter and McGoldrick (1989) proposed an eight-stage lifecycle to describe an individual's journey through family life:

- **Stage 1**
Live in family of origin with focus on relationships with parents and siblings, and have shared experiences.

- **Stage 2**
Leaving home, in which the individual establishes their own identity and creates a life beyond their family of origin.

- **Stage 3**

Pre-marriage stage, which involves developing long-term relationships and deciding to live together/get married.

- **Stage 4**

Childless couple stage, where couples develop ways of living together, become more influenced by their partner's extended family whilst loosening ties to their own family.

- **Stage 5**

Family with young children where the couple have to adjust their own relationship to accommodate the children's needs. Adults find their relationship with their own parents is reshaped. Children are initially completely family-oriented but start to develop relationships outside the immediate family.

- **Stage 6**

Family with adolescents. Children develop their autonomy and parent–child intimacy declines. Adults face mid-life issues regarding long-term relationships, and this is often the most demanding time in their working life.

- **Stage 7**

'Launching' children. Issues of loss for parents with children leaving and grandparents declining or dying, and reappraisal of their relationship as a childless couple. For children, the developing view of their parents as equals and ambivalence regarding their full independence.

- **Stage 8**

Later life, which involves adjustment to the effects of ageing for parents and possible loss of partner. For children the growth of responsibilities towards parents and death of their parents.

There are many obvious criticisms of this model, such as its assumption of couples staying together and the ability or desire to have children, as well as assumptions about culture and sexuality – which could be seen as a white Western stereotype – but the concept of an evolutionary process of family development is fairly universal, with most cultures and societies recognising the importance of the passage of significant milestones such as birth, puberty, marriage and death, usually marking them with ceremonies.

All cultures have expectations that inform the way families think about resolving disputes, the extent of involvement of the extended family, and how marriages and parent–child relationships should be conducted. It is also important to recognise that families exist in a broader context. For example a second generation family of Indian origin living in Britain may have different family expectations from the family of origin, as their family expectations could be a mixture of the differing influences. As with all developmental models there is danger that families come to be pathologised if they are not progressing to the next stage. Despite these criticisms, the family lifecycle model remains a useful framework for thinking about the family context in which young people develop, as it poses the question 'why is this family/young person presenting now?'

Young people often present with mental health problems at points of transition in the family lifecycle (Carter and McGoldrick 1989). A family that is appropriately equipped with strategies may still find transition difficult, but will be able to achieve the tasks necessary to make the transition successfully. A family that does not have the necessary skills or finds itself thrown off course by unexpected events may struggle to meet the tasks to enable a successful transition. Alongside the more predictable transitional stressors there is likely to be a range of factors that impinge on a family's ability to negotiate transitions between stages of the lifecycle. These can be unpredictable life events such as a premature death, illness, disability and

Case study: Nigel

Nigel is 17 years old and you have been asked to see him because he has complained of feeling increasingly anxious in social situations. He has also been losing interest in seeing his friends and struggling to keep up with his college work. He is an able student and hopes to go to university later this year. He gets on well with his parents, but his father recently had to retire due to a chronic heart condition. Nigel's older brother is in his second year at university. His maternal grandparents lived nearby and had always been fit and well, but his grandmother died last year and his grandfather needs a lot of support from Nigel's mother.

What lifecycle issues, both predictable and unpredictable, can you identify and how might they be affecting Nigel and the family?

redundancy. The parent's own experiences in their families of origin is a significant influence on how they approach the task of helping their children through difficult times. For example, a mother's ability to help her daughter negotiate the transition into adolescence may be seriously compromised by the unexpected loss of a parent when she was an adolescent. Carter and McGoldrick (1989) described these as horizontal and vertical stressors.

References

Carter, B. and McGoldrick, M. (1989) *The Changing Family Lifecycle: A Framework for Family Therapy* (2nd edition). New York: Gardner.

Levin, I. and Trost, J. (1992) 'Understanding the concept of family.' *Family Relations 41*, 348–351.

Office for National Statistics (2005) *Mental Health of Children and Young People in Great Britain, 2004.* Basingstoke: Palgrave McMillan.

Further reading

Carr, A. (2000) *Family Therapy: Concepts, Process and Practice.* Chichester: Wiley

Krause, I. and Miller, A.C. (1995) 'Culture and family therapy.' In S. Fernando (ed.) *Mental Health in a Multi-Ethnic Society: A Multidisciplinary Handbook.* London: Routledge.

McGoldrick, M., Pearce, J.K. and Giordana, J. (1996) *Ethnicity and Family Therapy* (2nd edition). New York: Guilford Press.

PART 3

Factors that Influence the Mental Health of Young People

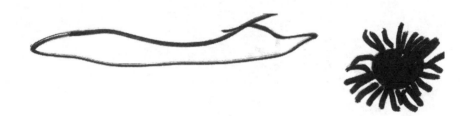

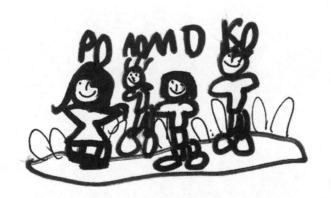

CHAPTER 6

What Causes Mental Health Problems in Young People?

There is no easy answer to this question. To answer it requires an understanding of all the factors that can play a part in causing mental health problems. Until recently those factors for which there were tangible interventions (such as family therapy, medication) were almost exclusively incorporated into theories to explain the causation (aetiology) of problems. For example, understanding a problem as being caused by how the family functions enables the professional to develop interventions based on improving family functioning. However, as this is a circular process, it can be difficult to evaluate the different components. Child mental health is now becoming a more evidence-based discipline, which means that theories of understanding causation and treatment are not necessarily based on the same assumptions.

So what causes child and adolescent mental health problems and disorders? Very few child and adolescent mental health problems are caused by a single factor; most are multifactorial in origin, that is several factors play a part in their development and often it may be the combination of factors that leads to problems. The impact of each factor varies from problem to problem and young person to young person. Traditionally there are three main areas that need consideration – biological, psychological and environmental – but whilst they are considered separately for clarity, it must be remembered that there is interaction between them all.

Biological factors

Biological factors refer to physical or physiological influences and may be inherited or acquired. They include:

- genetic (inheritance through one [single gene inheritance] or many [multiple gene inheritance] genes)

- chromosomal abnormalities (chromosomes are large packages of genetic material; any syndrome characterised by malformation or malfunction in any of the body's system may be caused by an abnormality in the number or structure of the chromosomes)

- developmental (e.g. malformations of the brain)

- medical disorders, especially neurological (affecting the brain and nervous system) or endocrine (hormonal)

- physical or chemical trauma (especially affecting the brain)

- metabolic disorders (causing e.g. biochemical imbalance)

- toxic disorders (substance use, heavy metals such as lead, and chemicals)

- dietary deficiencies (e.g. vitamins).

A similar range of categories may also cause developmental delay, though the specific factors involved may differ (see Chapter 4). Genetic and chromosomal factors may directly influence the development of a specific mental disorder, or their effect can be mediated by environmental factors. Physical abnormality or trauma to the brain is strongly associated with the development of mental health disorders, as are other disorders of the brain such as epilepsy. Other medical problems that may lead to mental health problems include:

- endocrine/hormonal (e.g. diabetes, thyroid dysfunction)

- infection

- chronic medical problems (e.g. cystic fibrosis, asthma)

- medication side-effects (e.g. steroids).

Specific medical problems are associated with particular presentations, for example hyperthyroidism (gives rise to raised levels of thyroxin) may cause anxiety; raised steroid levels (either owing to treatment or resulting from a primary endocrine disorder) may cause depression and aggression.

Developmental immaturity

There are also some presentations that are only defined as disorders should they continue beyond a certain age, for instance temper tantrums are common at age two or three, but are less common and acceptable at age six. By adolescence young people are expected to have attained greater control of their emotions.

Psychological factors
Attachment theory

Attachment theory was initially developed by Bowlby (1969, 1973) to try to understand how young people developed emotional links with their parents. Attachment is an adaptive biological process serving the needs of the child for protection and nurture. It is an interactive process, and though the attachment may be genetically determined, it is influenced by other factors (e.g. maternal mental health). It is of particular relevance in infancy, but features of attachment can be measured through childhood and into adulthood. The theory has been criticised as it centred on mothers, but it has relevance if the primary attachment figure (the person that the child has the closest attachment with, which is usually the primary caregiver) and other attachment figures are considered. The security of attachment is an important indicator of the quality of the parent–child relationship. Secure attachment predicts a better quality of the parent–child relationship in later years, as well as better skills at problem solving, increased cooperation, compliance and sharing of positive emotions by the child with the parent.

Deficiencies in the quantity and quality of contact with the main attachment figure can give rise to specific problems in the short term and long term. Bowlby (1980) later identified three stages in the short-term response by infants to separation from the attachment figure, known as the separation response. These were:

- Protest: the child is distressed, often crying and agitated, and may seek or call out for the attachment figure.

- Despair: the child expresses grief and misery at failure of the attachment figure to return, becoming listless with little interest and response to the immediate environment.

- Detachment: if the child enters this stage, the child may *appear* to have adapted and become content, and will show no interest when the attachment figure returns.

These findings and other studies of child deprivation influenced social policy on child welfare and many aspects of childcare over the following decade, for instance with the institution of parents sleeping in on paediatric wards. Previously, young people seen as 'troublesome' on separation from their parent(s) would later be reported – incorrectly – to have 'settled' as they reached the stage of detachment. Instead, priority is now given to maintaining contact of sufficient quality and duration in these circumstances.

PATTERNS OF ATTACHMENT

Ainsworth *et al.* (1978) described three main patterns of attachment that can be characterised by observation of the toddler's behaviour with the primary caregiver. These are based on the 12- to 20-month-old infant's reaction, in an experimental setting (known as the 'strange situation' procedure), over an 18-minute period to (a) exposure to a stranger while with the caregiver; (b) separation from the primary caregiver; (c) the return of the caregiver followed by departure of both; and (d) the return of the primary caregiver.

- **Secure attachment**
The primary caregiver provides a secure base for exploration, and the child is readily comforted if distressed. When reunited with the primary caregiver the child will seek and maintain contact if he/she has been distressed. The attachment is secure in that the child correctly anticipates that the primary caregiver will be there for them.

- **Anxious/resistant (clingy) attachment**
In this pattern of attachment the child is too anxious to leave the primary caregiver to explore his/her environment, and is more wary of new situations and people. When reunited after a separation the child

may be aggressive, cry and refuse to be comforted, or remain very passive and withdrawn.

•   Anxious/avoidant (detached) attachment
The child explores readily, often ignoring the primary caregiver. The child is unduly friendly with strangers. After separation the child will ignore or avoid the primary caregiver.

A fourth style of attachment has since been described, *disorganised*, in which the child demonstrates conflict behaviour, confusion, fear of the caregiver and unusual, repetitive, unproductive behaviours (Main and Solomon 1986).

It is important to emphasise that attachment disorder is not a diagnosis and is not a classification of the infant, but of the relationship. An infant will show different characteristics in their attachments to different people, and, for instance, with parents the nature of each attachment is predicted by that parent's characteristics. The nature of the attachment is not a reflection of the child's temperament. During the course of childhood, the characteristics of the child's attachments become more unified, such that by adolescence and adulthood an individual's pattern of social interaction is more integrated.

LONG-TERM CONSEQUENCES

Theories based on the importance of relationships in the first five years of life predict that early separation from attachment figures leads to poor outcomes in later childhood and adulthood. However, earlier studies of the long-term effects of separation are contradictory. Some studies confirmed this prediction, for example young people raised in institutions had higher rates of behaviour problems, related to adults with 'attention-seeking' or 'clingy' behaviour, and were less attached to their mothers on return. However, young people from disrupted homes and young people adopted later in childhood had largely good outcomes, which depended on several factors and not solely early life experiences. Case studies of young people with profound deprivation (such as complete lack of contact with others, being locked in cupboards for prolonged periods) established that over a period of time with appropriate parenting they were able to catch up in their development and function normally at home and school.

Personality, temperament and self-identity

The psychological makeup of an individual, including their personality, may play a part in the development of mental health problems, so that a young person who has an anxiety trait may be more at risk of developing generalised anxiety or depression. An individual with a penchant for perfection may be at greater risk of developing obsessive-compulsive disorder. This is often also a reason why young people who have experienced similar events may cope very differently.

How others perceive us and the concept of 'who I am' are important to child mental health because of their links with behaviour, emotion states and cognitions. Humans are essentially social, so our definition of self is necessarily in the context of relations with others, though the degree to which people see themselves as independent (or as individuals) varies between cultures. In Eastern societies there tends to be a greater emphasis on self in the context of the family and society, whereas in Western societies the emphasis is more on individualism.

The following terms will be used in this section, and their generally accepted definitions are:

- *Personality*: The totality of predisposing behavioural tendencies that is an identifiable ingrained pattern of response. Personality is not normally considered to be fully developed until late adolescence.

- *Traits*: Circumscribed aspects of personality (i.e. one's predictable behavioural response to a given event/situation).

- *Temperament*: Components of personality for which there is an implied genetic contribution, further influenced by parental attitudes and child-rearing practices.

CHARACTERISTICS OF PERSONALITY

The words *personality* and *character* are often incorrectly used interchangeably. Personality refers to the whole pattern of psychological function, whilst character refers to distinguishing qualities. The concept of 'the whole' as being greater than the identifiable parts applies to personality, which confounds attempts to measure it. As with physical characteristics, we all differ, and yet share many qualities.

Personality and personality traits are much more useful concepts in adult mental health. In young people personality is not fully formed, and it is more helpful to refer to specific 'building blocks' of personality, known as temperament.

CHARACTERISTICS OF TEMPERAMENT

Temperament is probably inherited through many genes (polygenic), and there are also environmental influences. However, twin studies suggest that environmental influences lessen with time. Temperament is enduring, showing continuity throughout childhood.

In contrast to the assessment of personality in adults, which is largely based on self-report, the assessment of temperament relies on observers. The people likely to have the most complete set of observations and experiences of the child are usually parents. However, there are difficulties in relying on parental report of temperament because of the influence of factors such as the quality of the parent–child relationship, beliefs held by the wider family ('family myths'), and possibly the parents' relationship.

Nine categories of temperamental attributes have been identified: activity level, rhythmicity, approach/withdrawal, adaptability, threshold of responsiveness, intensity of reaction, quality of mood, distractibility, and attention span /persistence. The sum of these characteristics leads to a simple three-way classification of young people's temperament as 'easy', 'difficult', or 'slow-to-warm-up'. Most young people are described as having an easy temperament and this provides a relative protection against psychological problems. Difficult temperament predisposes to behavioural/conduct problems. Slow-to-warm-up temperament predisposes to emotional problems. However, these observations are limited by reliance on parent report, difficulty defining onset of a specific disorder (and thus distinguishing pre-existing factors from characteristics of the disorder), difficulties measuring specific characteristics (such as impulsivity), and interaction with environmental factors.

There is an interaction between the child's temperament and their emotional environment. 'Goodness of fit' describes a concept of how favourable this interaction is (Thomas and Chess 1977). A particularly important aspect of this is the interaction between the child and the parent: a dynamic pattern of behaviour is established and is prone to repetition.

The parent's behaviour in response to the child's behaviour influences the child's next behaviour, which in turn influences the parent's next behaviour, and so on.

SELF-IDENTITY

Self-identity, or how we conceive of ourselves, is commonly considered to have two components. Self-image is the factual account of ourselves in physical terms (such as height, weight, etc.) and psychological traits (such as likes and dislikes). Self-esteem is the personal judgement of the quality and value of these traits, and the worth of oneself as a person.

SELF-IMAGE

The assessment of our own factual traits may lead us to conclude that we differ significantly from the social group to which we belong. This may be on the basis of behaviour, beliefs, physical appearance, ability, sexuality, sexual orientation, ethnicity or other characteristics. This may or may not affect self-esteem. It may lead to attempts to modify those traits, modify the social group or change group. Self-image may also be distorted, for example distortions of the concept of one's own physical size and shape are core features of anorexia nervosa.

SELF-ESTEEM

Self-esteem has been studied since the late 1960s, when a simple classification based on quantification (high, medium, and low) was found to correlate with behaviour. When boys were studied, those boys with high self-esteem were physically fitter, and more active, expressive, ambitious and successful. Boys with low self-esteem were more likely to experience headaches, insomnia and stomach complaints. There are also gender differences in attribution in that girls attribute negative events to themselves and positive events to other influences (either the environment or factors such as luck), whilst boys do the reverse. Young people with high self-esteem are more likely to have involved parents, who are clear and firm at setting limits and have higher expectations of their child. Self-esteem in turn can influence patterns of thinking, and with more likelihood of identifying failure there may be a relationship with the development of disorders such as depression.

We learn about ourselves through the relationships that we have with others, and this is true from early infancy. Our concept of 'self' changes with the constantly changing nature of these relationships and the experiences we have. We learn more about ourselves from each new experience. This is of great importance in childhood, with relatively fewer experiences on which to base the concept of self. Increased autonomy accompanies the child's growth of the concept. The development of relationships and the development of the concept of self may be two sides of the same coin.

Psychoanalytical factors

These derive from the work of Freud but have been developed further by Anna Freud, Klein and many others. Some of the theories developed by Eriksen and Bowlby have transformed psychoanalytical theory so that they now have only a tenuous link with Freud's original ideas.

One of the biggest strengths of Freud's work was the development of the concept of defence mechanisms – that is strategies that individuals use to cope with difficult situations or feelings. There are several defence mechanisms. One example is projection, in which one's own unacceptable thoughts or feelings are transferred to another person. So instead of acknowledging one's own anger, an individual may state that someone else is angry. Displacement is another commonly used defence mechanism where aggression or anger is transferred from the real issue to another. Most people use defence mechanisms at some time or another, their use is only a problem if they continue to be used as a long-term measure, thus preventing the resolution of issues that may cause conflict.

Behavioural theories

Behavioural theories assert that behaviour and emotional expression are learned as a result of experience. Four theories predominate.

- **Classical conditioning**

First described by Pavlov (1927), this involves the repeated introduction of a neutral stimulus alongside one that is known to induce a physiological or behavioural response – until the neutral stimulus alone induces the same response, and is then known as the conditioned stimulus.

- **Operant conditioning**

First described by Skinner (1953), this is a process whereby the frequency of behaviour is influenced by its consequences. A behaviour becomes more frequent if it commonly leads to a reward (positive reinforcement), or avoidance of an undesirable or unpleasant consequence (negative reinforcement). A behaviour becomes less frequent if it commonly leads to no reward (extinction), or an undesirable or unpleasant consequence (punishment). Of these four, positive reinforcement and extinction are the most influential on the frequency of behaviour. Positive reinforcement is more potent when it is intermittent and irregular.

- **Social learning theory**

First described by Bandura (1977), this emphasises the importance of human relationships in behaviour and the observations people make of each other. In this way, vicarious experience leads to learning – a process known as modelling. Participant modelling, in which the person also actively takes part, has the highest learning rate. Patterson (1982) described the dynamic interplay between parent and child as each influences the other's behaviour. These findings, which were the result of systematic observation of parent–child interactions, have influenced the development of family behavioural interventions over the last two to three decades and informed the further exploration of the parent–child relationship.

- **Cognitive learning**

This underpins cognitive-behavioural approaches and recognises the importance of cognitions that accompany behaviour, which may be generally positive (e.g. self-congratulatory) or negative (e.g. self-denigratory). Cognitive learning theory regards learning as a process of thinking about and understanding behaviours and of consciously seeking solutions to problems, rather than seeing acquired behaviours as a series of unconscious responses to environmental stimuli.

Environmental factors

Social theory states that the young person's environment plays a part in the development of their problems. Environment may include the family, school, peer group, community, and life-events such as bereavement, road accidents, and so on. Young people on the margins of normative or cultural (in the very broadest sense) groups may also be at increased risk of developing mental health problems.

Family theories

For young people, the family (or the lack of it) plays a key role in their development. Family theories conceptualise that processes and communications that go on within families may result in the development of problems within the family. These problems may be presented through the identification of a problem in one family member, who is usually a child. Sibling order can also play a part in the development of some problems although the reasons for this are not clear. In clinic samples, young people who live in families under stress are more likely to be referred than young people with the same level of problems who live in well-functioning families.

STYLES OF PARENTING

Young people's need for affection and control is well established. These qualities have been described in families in terms of parenting style (Carr 2000; Darling and Steinberg 1993). Using these two qualities it is possible to describe four different styles of parenting and the likely outcomes for young people subjected to these styles.

1. **Authoritative parenting**

   When parents combine lots of warmth with a degree of control. This tends to provide the most beneficial environment for a child's emotional development.

2. **Permissive parenting**

   When parents are warm and accepting of their children but exert little control on their behaviour. These children often fail to develop sufficient self-control and problem-solving skills.

3. **Authoritarian parenting**

   When parents are warm but overcontrolling and overinvolved. These young people develop a way of interacting with the world that avoids conflict and demonstrates little initiative.

4. Neglecting parenting

When a lack of parental warmth is combined with control, which is sometimes harsh but always inconsistent. This style is associated with the worst outcomes for young people and can be a significant factor leading to their presentation with mental health problems in childhood and adolescence.

These styles can develop from the parents' own experience of being parented and can result from differing parental beliefs about child rearing, parental relationship difficulties, parental mental health problems (such as depression, which can cause the parent to feel emotionally detached and lacking in motivation) or as a reaction or response to a temperamentally difficult child.

FAMILY LIFECYCLE EVENTS

A family's difficulty in negotiating the transition between the stages of the family lifecycle (as described earlier) can often be a point at which a child presents with mental health problems. What seems to make a difference at these transitions is a family's level of flexibility. The family's ability to manage change and the perceptions of individuals about the family vary at different stages. For example, this ability begins to decline as young people enter adolescence and reaches its lowest point just as young people are preparing to leave home.

FAMILY STRUCTURE CHANGES

Changes in family structure may result from death of a family member, separation, divorce, fostering and adoption. Structural changes in families are an increasingly common experience for young people, therefore it is important to consider the consequences for them of these events. Generally speaking, if the parental relationship is chronically acrimonious, irrespective of whether the parents stay together or separate, the impact on the young people will be considerable. This impact is compounded if young people are caught up in continuing hostility and its consequences. The age at which the young person experiences the separation will also influence the different issues that young people may face as a result of parental separation or divorce.

It is virtually impossible to disentangle the effect of separation from the effect of socio-economic disadvantage (Wadsby 1993) as the two are so closely linked in the UK. The experiences in countries where the socio-economic effect of separation is lessened by a more generous welfare and benefit system suggest that many of the negative effects associated with separation (such as poorer mental health outcomes) are linked more to social disadvantage than to the emotional turmoil. This view, however, is contradicted to some extent in other studies (Amato 1993).

Rodgers and Pryor's (1998) wide-ranging review of outcome studies points to a strong association between parental separation and conduct disorders in young people and an association with higher levels of distress and unhappiness. Most studies suggest that this effect is temporary and begins to fall after 18 months to 2 years. With adolescents and young adults there is good evidence of a relationship between parental separation and mental health problems and substance abuse. The link between parental separation and a higher risk of depressive symptoms in adolescence is well established in UK studies.

The experience of losing a parent through death increases the likelihood of behavioural problems in young people and adolescents. However, taken overall the impact is less than that of a child experiencing parental separation especially when considering the longer-term mental health consequences. Stepfamilies also have long- and short-term implications for young people and young people's mental health. While re-partnering can go some way to lessen the socio-economic effects of separation and single parenthood, many of the protective factors for families and young people are reduced with attendant risks for the child and the adult relationship. Most difficulties in relationships and adjustment to transitions in stepfamilies occur when young people are in early adolescence. When compared with single parent families, on the other hand, children tend to fare better in stepfamilies.

Overall it is the experience of multiple changes in family structure that significantly increases the likelihood of adverse outcomes. Young people of separated families are more likely to experience these multiple changes because of the greater chances of subsequent parental relationships breaking down.

Peer influences

Whilst the importance of a warm and positive relationship with a significant adult is widely acknowledged, the development of social relationships outside the family from middle childhood onwards is a significant protective factor in young people's mental health. The ability to make and keep friends can counter extremely adverse experiences. With young people who survived concentration camps in the Second World War, those who had developed strong peer relationships demonstrated far better mental health outcomes.

Young people who fail to develop friendships and acquire some skills in peer relationships are at greater risk of developing mental health problems in adolescence and early adulthood. Peer relationships are where most young people learn about managing conflict and early peer interaction is important for the development of self-esteem and a child's sense of place in the wider world. Unpopular young people often get caught up in a pattern of poor peer relationships because of their limited social skills and fixed models of interacting with their peers; as a consequence unpopularity is often a long-term experience. Two types of unpopular child are identified by Carr (2000): the aggressive, disruptive child and the sensitive, anxious, often bullied child. This pattern has been noted across several cultures and both types have been shown to have low self-esteem. Carr estimates that 10–15 per cent of young people could be described as unpopular and are rejected by their peer group.

In adolescence, peer culture has been shown to have a strong influence, both positive and negative, on educational outcomes, which in turn is a clear factor in young people's mental health. However, there is evidence that peer influences are not merely accidental and that there is a large degree of choice about peer group selection. By the age of 12–14 in Western societies there is a sharp decline in the young person's choice of a parent as the primary confidant and a marked preference for peers. The desire to conform to the peer group peaks around the ages of 13 and 14. Both of these factors are important considerations when working with young people and mental health.

Impact of school

School plays a big part in young people's lives. It is often the first exposure to the world outside the family, which for many children will begin with nursery school. The way children settle into this environment is a good predictor of longer-term outcomes. Those children that have peer difficulties or behavioural problems are likely to continue to have them in later years unless the problems are addressed. For most young people school is a positive experience. For many though it can be a very difficult environment, either because they struggle with the work or because the environment is too challenging for them. To function well in school, young people need to be able to tolerate rules and boundaries as well as sustain relationships with peers and adults. They may also have to cope with stressors such as bullying. It is well recognised that young people who struggle with their schoolwork are at increased risk of behavioural problems. There can be a tendency to focus on the behaviour rather than consider why the child is struggling.

Young people with neurological disorders, including epilepsy, are particularly vulnerable to failing in school. Failing in school impacts negatively on self-esteem and self-confidence. It also means that young people miss out on developing appropriate peer relationships. An educational psychologist should be the first point of contact for school staff who have concerns about a young person's educational progress or behaviour problems. The educational psychologist can then assess the young person to clarify whether he or she has a learning disability or specific learning problems. It is usually necessary for the young person's cognitive ability to be assessed. The psychologist, school staff and parents can then work together to develop the best strategies to help the young person.

Schools can impact positively on young people by providing them with a supportive and challenging environment. A positive relationship with a teacher can mitigate the impact of less positive experiences. School exams and coursework can generate stress in young people, and it is important that they are helped to address this as they are likely to come across it again in their lives. Schools should consider addressing it in a proactive way through the development of workshops that help young people recognise their stress and deal with it appropriately. Schools are also well placed to enhance social development through 'buddy' systems and 'circle of friends' in the classroom in younger children, and the use of social skills groups in older children and adolescents.

The impact of culture

Defining culture is difficult. Each individual has their own assigned meaning of culture. For some it is defined by skin colour, religion or racial background; for others country of origin, sexuality, and so on. It is likely to be a combination of all of these with some aspects playing a more dominant part than others. Whatever group an individual may belong to, they remain unique because of their experiences and interpretations of their experiences.

Studies in the UK have found that in Gujarati preschool children there may be less psychological disturbance than in peers from a non-Gujarati background. It is possible that there is no difference in the behaviours of the children, but what is culturally bound is the parental responses to the behaviours. For example, Gujarati parents may tolerate different levels of non-compliance than their English counterparts. However, whether this is changing, as second and third generation individuals become parents, remains to be seen.

Culture strongly influences the role of parents and of young people. Whilst traditional domestic routines may continue to be of great importance to young people of British minority ethnic groups growing up in the UK, this is not seen as the only way to do things and they are increasingly exposed to other cultures. South Asian young people may be brought up with a strong sense of family responsibility implicit in particular relationships. The role of brother/sister, son/daughter, maternal uncle/paternal aunt involve particular duties and privileges (Jackson and Nesbitt 1993). However, in wider society they are exposed to different expectations. Where there is a tendency for the family to have a central role, the needs of the family and the needs of the individual may conflict. Asian girls, and especially those who find their choices restricted because of cultural expectations, can experience considerable distress. This can be compounded by the unwillingness of minority groups to discuss this openly. However, culture can also provide young people with a sense of belonging and some appreciation of their role.

Less research has been undertaken on African-Caribbean young people in the UK. It is however, clear that African-Caribbean young people are more likely to be excluded from school than all other groups and more likely to get caught up in the criminal justice system. It is possible that being excluded from school, and the attendant risks associated with that, is a more significant factor than being African-Caribbean. Adult mental health still struggles to answer questions of whether professionals are more likely to attribute mental health diagnoses to African-Caribbean individuals than to other races. This is a question that child mental health has not yet begun to address.

American studies have investigated the help-seeking behaviour in African-American, Latino and Caucasian youth. Minority parents appeared more reluctant to access services. This may be for several reasons, including concerns that they will not be understood, previous experience, and differing cultural interpretations of behaviours and methods to manage them. However, services for young people may need to engage these populations more actively.

The impact of the community

There is a higher prevalence of mental health problems in economically disadvantaged areas and in communities where there is a lack of a stable population. Support networks in these communities tend to be poorly developed. Urbanisation of society has led to changes in community structures. National crime rates tend to be positively correlated with the proportion of the population in urban residence. Young people may find themselves at increased risk of being involved in crime, both as perpetrators and victims. Urbanisation is also associated with an increased differential between living standards of the affluent and the poor, and increased residential segregation by class and minority group. The

Case study: Leanne

Leanne was an 11-year-old whose mother had been diagnosed with breast cancer several months earlier. Leanne's family had told her that her mother was 'poorly' but had sought to protect her from the details of the extensive treatment her mother had to undergo. This was now complete and Leanne's mother's progress was very positive. Previously Leanne had been getting on well at school and had an active social life, but over the past two months she had been increasingly reluctant to go to school and leave the house. This culminated with a complete school refusal at the move to secondary school and several episodes of acute anxiety when Leanne's father tried to get her to go to school.

economically disadvantaged areas have larger schools and bigger classes, with less parental involvement than wealthier areas. This may result in poor education, and especially affected will be those with special educational needs. There may also be increased exposure to violence (both domestic and non-domestic), discrimination and parental mental health problems (related to issues of stress). All of these factors are interrelated and can significantly impact on the development of mental health problems in young people. However, for some young people, urbanisation can offer diversification of educational and recreational opportunities.

References

Ainsworth, M.D.S., Blehar, M., Waters, E. and Wall, S. (1978) *Patterns of Attachment: A Psychological Study of the Strange Situation.* Hillsdale, NJ: Lawrence Erlbaum Associates.

Amato, P.R. (1993) 'Children's adjustments to divorce: Theories, hypotheses and empirical support.' *Journal of Marriage and the Family 55,* 23–28.

Bandura, A. (1977) *Social Learning Theory.* Englewood Cliffs, NJ: Prentice-Hall.

Bowlby, J. (1969) *Attachment and Loss. Vol.1: Attachment.* London: Hogarth Press.

Bowlby, J. (1973) *Attachment and Loss. Vol.2: Separation: Anxiety and Anger.* London: Hogarth Press.

Bowlby, J. (1980) *Attachment and Loss. Vol.3: Loss: Sadness and Depression.* London: Hogarth Press.

Carr, A. (2000) *Family Therapy: Concepts, Process and Practice.* Chichester: Wiley.

Darling, N. and Steinberg, L. (1993) 'Parenting style as context: An integrative model.' *Psychological Bulletin 113,* 487–496.

Jackson, R. and Nesbitt, E. (1993) *Hindu Children in Britain.* Stoke on Trent, England: Trentham Books.

Main, M. and Solomon, J. (1986) 'Discovery of an insecure disorganized/disorientated attachment pattern: Procedures, findings and implications for the development of behaviour.' In M. Yogman and T.B. Brazelton (eds) *Affective Development in Infancy.* Norwood, NJ: Ablex.

Patterson, G.R. (1982) *Coercive Family Process.* Eugene, OR: Castalia.

Pavlov, I.P. (1927) *Conditioned Reflexes* (translated by G.V. Anrep). Oxford: Clarendon Press.

Rodgers, B. and Pryor, J. (1998) *Divorce and Separation: The Outcomes for Children.* York: Joseph Rowntree Foundation.

Skinner, B.F. (1953) *Science and Human Behaviour.* New York: Macmillan.

Thomas, A. and Chess, S. (1977) *Temperament and Development.* New York: Brunner/Mazel.

Wadsby, M. (1993) *Children of Divorce and their Parents.* Linkoping University medical dissertations, Number 405. Linkoping: Linkoping University.

Further reading

Helman, C.G. (2000) *Culture, Health and Illness: An Introduction for Health Professionals* (4th edition). Abingdon: Bookpoint.

Main, M. (1996) 'Overview of the field of attachment.' *Journal of Consulting and Clinical Psychology 64,* 237–243.

Parkes, C.M. and Stevenson-Hinde, J. (1982) *The Place of Attachment in Human Behaviour.* London: Tavistock Publications.

Parkes, C.M., Stevenson-Hinde, J. and Marris, P. (1991) *Attachment Across the Life Cycle.* London: Routledge.

Rutter, M. (ed.) (1995) *Psychosocial Disturbances in Young People: Challenges for Prevention.* Cambridge: Press Syndicate of the University of Cambridge.

Steinhausen, H-C. and Verhulst, F. (1999) *Risks and Outcomes in Developmental Psychopathology.* Oxford: Oxford University Press.

CHAPTER 7

Protective and Adverse Factors Relating to Child Mental Health

Introduction

There is evidence that some factors or characteristics are likely to lead to an increase in mental health problems whilst some protect against the development of problems. Unfortunately, it is still not known how protective factors work. It is likely to be a complex relationship between an individual and their environment. It is useful to be aware of protective factors as primary care staff can try to ensure they are in place or maximised to enable young people to break the cycles of poverty, deprivation and mental health problems related to the environment.

There are groups of young people who are more likely to experience mental health problems. However, this does not mean that all young people from these groups experience problems.

Protective factors

Generally protective factors include:

- High intellectual ability and academic success, which give the young person opportunities to focus on long-term goals and build up a positive self-image. Academic success is often also seen as a way out of poverty and may present greater opportunities.

- Easy temperament as described in Chapter 6.

- Developing a warm and confiding relationship with a trustworthy and reliable adult (not necessarily within the family). This enables the young person to develop a support mechanism as well as developing trust with an adult.

- Having special skills or a particular talent (sporting or musical talents may be especially useful in giving young people opportunities to leave difficult circumstances behind).

- Peer relationships and friendships. Adults can often underestimate the support that young people provide for each other, especially during adolescence. Positive peer relationships give young people an opportunity to share their concerns and consider alternative ways of managing stress or difficulties. Peer relationships also enable young people to have fun.

- A supportive family that is able to manage change.

FAMILY RESILIENCE

Just as factors can lead to resilience in young people, there are factors that can indicate a family's level of resilience. Highlighting and developing a family's strengths can promote a more collaborative way of working with the family compared with earlier ideas of dysfunctional families.

What explains the different outcomes for families who have broadly similar experiences? First, a family's ability both to maintain its core structures, strengths and values and at the same time to balance this with a capacity to develop new patterns and structures flexibly. Second, the way families interpret or ascribe meaning to events is an indicator of their resilience. Connected with this is a family's ability to contemplate alternative perspectives to a given event. Studies of families who have experienced divorce suggest better outcomes for those that have a coherent family 'story' about the breakdown of the marriage and responsibilities both before and after the divorce. Third, Olson (1988) identified what he termed 'critical family resources', which enable families to weather periods of stress. These resources varied to some extent across the family lifecycle but broadly speaking can be identified as:

- parental relationship strengths, such as good communication, financial management and a mutually satisfactory sexual relationship

- family accord
- the subjective experience of satisfaction with the couple relationship and quality of family life.

Adverse factors

Adverse factors include:

External to the individual

- lack of stable placement
- lack of appropriate parenting
- parental illness (especially mental illness)
- domestic violence
- experiencing abuse (physical, sexual or emotional)
- low socio-economic status.

Individual factors

- poor strategies to cope with stress or difficulty
- poor educational attainment
- poor peer relationships
- developmental delay
- physical health problems.

Vulnerable young people who have experienced or face adversity

Young people who have experienced or face adversity are at increased risk of developing mental health problems and are often considered to be vulnerable. They are considered to be vulnerable because they have certain attributes or have had past or present experiences, or they are growing up in the face of adversity. Sometimes they may have a combination of attributes or experiences (Vostanis 2007). Young people from these vulnerable groups are some of the most disturbed and distressed young people in society. Their problems often stay with them into their adult lives and may re-emerge when they themselves become parents.

In addition, vulnerable young people can also experience a number of challenges that can exacerbate the complexity of their needs. These challenges can include the experience of increased stigma, movement of their location and displacement, difficulties in communicating their needs and having them understood, poor and unstable living conditions and school circumstances, and being subject to violence, abuse or even disaster.

Young people may often be given incomplete explanations of what is happening around them, thus compounding their difficulties. Adverse factors do not lead to a specific mental health problem but increase general vulnerability to experiencing problems. They can also face difficulties in accessing services that are appropriate to their needs. The best way for professionals to provide services that are responsive to these young people's needs is to provide them through close working partnerships, thus ensuring collaborative approaches that do not allow young people to slip through gaps in provision (Vostanis 2007).

It is important to emphasise that not all young people in these at-risk groups will experience mental health problems. Some show 'resilience' and have sufficient protective factors. It may be that even during such complex and difficult life circumstances, young people will be able to have enduring friendships, achieve educationally or have some life experiences that still offer some stability, for instance regular communication with a relative or stability within the school environment.

Groups of young people at high risk of developing mental health problems are highlighted here so professionals are better able to consider the needs of these young people. Some young people may belong to more than one group.

Young people who have experienced abuse

The numbers of young people who have experienced physical, sexual or emotional abuse, or a combination of these vary dependent on the definition of abuse. It is difficult to obtain figures for sexual abuse as much of it may not be disclosed until adulthood; and figures for emotional abuse are even less reliable as much of it is not even identified. It is suggested that in the UK approximately 10 per cent of young people have been sexually abused. The response of adults to disclosure of abuse may affect how young people themselves cope with the issues. Young people may find that disclosure of abuse may lead to retribution against them in the form of further abuse. They may find themselves in care and may perceive this as a punishment.

Young people in care

There are over 50,000 young people in the care of local authorities in England and Wales at any one time, and in the UK this group is currently called 'children looked after'. Around 18,000 of these young people live in residential units and community placements (National Children's Bureau 1998). There is evidence to show that looked-after young people have complex health and social needs, including higher rates of mental health problems. Their needs may be significantly higher with between 60 and 80 per cent having significant mental health problems and requiring specialist treatment, which is often lacking.

Young people who are homeless

It is difficult to be sure of the numbers of young people who are homeless as the definition of homelessness varies. However, a significant number of these young people are also likely to have been in care. They have often witnessed domestic violence, experienced abuse, have substance use problems, or have unmet mental health needs. In addition to homeless families with young people, there will be adolescents who are living in temporary hostels or living on the streets.

Young offenders

The needs of this group are not dissimilar to those of the looked-after group in that these young people often also have multiple and complex needs. Young offenders have significantly higher rates than their non-offending peers of serious mental illness, problem substance use, educational failure, past abuse, which has often been more persistent and deviant than that experienced by other abused young people, and social isolation or deviant peer contact (Kroll 2004). Many of these needs are not recognised by professionals working with them, and even when recognised they can be difficult to address. There are worryingly high rates of suicide and self-harm by young people in custody. There can be a reluctance by professionals to accept that these young people should be entitled to the same level of services as other young people, which coupled with young people's own ambivalence can be difficult to overcome.

Young people excluded from school

These young people already have significant problems, which led to their exclusion from school. Exclusion compounds the problems of poor peer relationships and poor educational achievement. These young people are at increased risk of becoming involved in crime as well as developing mental health problems.

Young people with physical disorders

Young people with physical disorders, including neurological conditions, have mental health problems more often than physically healthy young people. The rates of mental health problems in an Isle of Wight study were 7 per cent for physically well young people, 12 per cent for young people with physical disorders and 34 per cent for young people with brain disorders including epilepsy. Disorders of emotion and conduct were more common in the epilepsy sample and severity of central nervous system damage was a better predictor of developing mental health problems than site of damage. Many of the physically ill young people without a neurological condition had levels of functional disability similar to those with epilepsy, but they had lower rates of mental health problems. This may indicate that brain damage plays an important aetiological role, although the nature of the damage may be difficult to identify (Rutter, Tizard and Wightmore 1970). The support available to young people with epilepsy may also influence their emotional adjustment and management of the disorder. Recent studies have found that young people with physical health problems continue to have higher rates of mental health problems (Cadman *et al.* 1987; Gortmaker *et al.* 1990; Office for National Statistics 2005).

Young people who are refugees or asylum seekers

Young refugees or asylum seekers are at high risk of developing mental health problems. These may be related to the reasons for leaving their home (such as witnessing or experiencing violence and other atrocities, guilt about surviving when others did not, bereavement, and loss of contact with family) or related to settling into a new community (such as isolation, lack of access to positive aspects of their culture, racism and discrimination, poor housing, poverty and parents under stress).

References

Cadman, D., Boyle, M., Szatmaris, P. and Offord, D. (1987) 'Chronic illness, disability and mental and social well being: Findings of the Ontario Child Health Study.' *Paediatrics 79*, 5, 805–812.

Gortmaker, S.L., Walker, D.K., Weitzman, M. and Sobol, A.M. (1990) 'Chronic conditions, socioeconomic risks, and behavioural problems in children and adolescents.' *Paediatrics 85*, 3, 267–276.

Kroll, L. (2004) 'Needs assessment in adolescent offenders.' In S. Bailey and M. Dolan (eds) *Adolescent Forensic Psychiatry*. London: Arnold.

National Children's Bureau (1998) *Review of the Gatsby Investment in 'Young People Living in Public Care'*. London: National Young People's Bureau, Young People's Residential Care Unit 1996–1998.

Olson, D. (1988) 'Family types, family stress and family satisfaction: A family development perspective.' In C. Falicor (ed.) *Family Transitions*. New York: Guilford Press.

Office of National Statistics (2005) The Mental Health of Children and Young people in Great Britain, 2004. Basingstoke: Palgrave McMillan.

Rutter, M., Tizard, J. and Wightmore, K. (1970) *Education, Health and Behaviour*. London: Longman.

Vostanis, P. (ed.) (2007) *Mental Health Services and Interventions for Vulnerable Children and Young People*. London: Jessica Kingsley Publishers.

Further reading

Hester, M., Pearson, C. and Harwin, N. (2000) *Making an Impact: Children and Domestic Violence – A Reader*. London: Jessica Kingsley Publishers.

Hinde, R. and Stevenson-Hinde, J. (1988) *Relationships within Families: Mutual Influences*. Oxford: Clarendon Press.

Jackson, S. and Thomas, N. (2000) *What Works in Creating Stability for Looked After Children* (2nd edition). Ilford, Essex: Barnardo's.

Kurtz, Z. (1996) *Treating Young People Well*. London: Mental Health Foundation.

McGee, C. (2000) *Childhood Experiences of Domestic Violence*. London: Jessica Kingsley Publishers.

Richardson, J. and Joughin, C. (2000) *The Mental Health Needs of Looked After Children*. Focus College Research Unit. London: Gaskell.

Rutter, M. (ed.) (1995) *Psychosocial Disturbances in Young People: Challenges for Prevention*. Cambridge: Press Syndicate of the University of Cambridge.

Vostanis, P. and Cumella, S. (eds) (1999) *Homeless Children: Problems and Needs*. London: Jessica Kingsley Publishers.

PART 4

Specific Mental Health Problems of Childhood and Adolescence

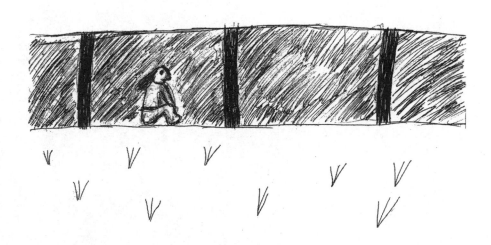

CHAPTER 8

Emotional Problems

Defining emotional problems

'Emotional disorder of childhood' has commonly been used as an all-embracing term for the variety of emotional problems with which young people can present. The reasons for such a broad category have been that:

- presentations vary with age and development

- young people often present with a mixture of symptoms that include significant changes in the young person's mood, changes in behaviour, and physical symptoms

- the mixture of symptoms (i.e. their presence and relative significance) varies considerably between young people, to a point that makes further categorisation potentially complex.

Despite these issues, different types of emotional problem have recently been more clearly distinguished, and these are usually defined on the predominant change in mood. These may include anxiety, worry, fear, sadness, misery, depression and anger. Anger does not usually feature as a mental health problem but is included here as intervention is often made with young people to help emotional or social development.

The next question in defining emotional problems is, 'When is a problem a problem?' There are two aspects to the young person's presentation that are helpful in defining this: first, whether the symptoms cause the young person (or others) a significant degree of distress, and second, whether the symptoms have an adverse effect on social or educational function. A third factor may be assessed in longer-term issues: that of the effect on the young person's psychological or physical development. The case of Richard (below) describes features that are helpful in determining the distress caused to him and the impact of his symptoms on function and potentially on development.

Case study: Richard

Richard is an 11-year-old boy who was seen by his school nurse after he was reported by his teacher to be tearful on a number of occasions in playtime and after school. Over two appointments Richard began to describe how he feels worried at night, often cries himself to sleep, has nightmares about his family being in a car accident and on two occasions has had panic attacks. He is tired a lot, finds it difficult to concentrate on his schoolwork, and is particularly upset with himself because he 'just can't be bothered to do things any more' – despite being very conscientious normally. He thinks this is all 'silly' and can no longer face playing with his friends because he is afraid of what they might think of him. He has managed to hide it from his parents, thinking that they would tell him off.

Richard was first upset watching a TV programme two months ago about how stress might cause cancer, which is what his grandfather died of a few weeks before that. He was very close to his grandfather, who had given Richard some good advice on lots of things. Richard had even wondered whether he was a stress to his grandfather and therefore caused his death. This thought was very painful and kept coming back to him – 'even in class'.

What should the school nurse also enquire about?

How should Richard's concern about telling his parents be approached?

What specific interventions should be made?

Types of emotional disorder

There are two broad groups of emotional disorders – anxiety disorders and depressive disorders. In addition, there are some disorders that are partly defined by an identified precipitant, such as adjustment reaction, abnormal bereavement reaction and posttraumatic stress disorder. Depression is covered in Chapter 12.

Anxiety and anxiety disorders

Anxiety serves a biological function in ensuring survival, which is mediated by a number of observed mechanisms such as attachment, learning, physiological response, and avoidance of danger. The degree to which we experience and use anxiety is influenced by our genetic inheritance, temperament and life experiences. Anxiety can become habitually maladaptive, causing distress and dysfunction, at which point it may be defined as a disorder. There is a high prevalence of reported anxiety in population studies, but a relatively low presentation in clinics, which implies that most anxiety-related problems are tolerated and do not cause significant dysfunction. This may partly explain the many and varied definitions to distinguish an anxiety disorder from the normal experience of anxiety.

Anxiety disorders may present in young people in a variety of ways. Some are situation-specific and some are general. The four most common anxiety disorders in young people are separation anxiety, phobic disorders, social anxiety and generalised anxiety (previously called overanxious disorder). Panic disorder can also present in childhood.

Features of anxiety disorders include affective, cognitive and physical (or somatic) components. Affective features necessarily include a subjective experience of anxiety, which may be reported – especially in younger children – as fear, scared feelings, being afraid or worry. Young people also commonly report misery, sadness and sometimes anger, when it is important to exclude depressive disorders. Cognitive features may include the belief that self or a family member is at risk of death or illness, that an event has occurred or will occur as a result of the young person's own action (or inaction), and fear of imminent (though not necessarily definable) disaster. Somatic features include headaches, stomach aches, shortness of breath, a choking sensation, pins and needles in hands or feet, dry mouth, blurred vision, a repeated sense of the need to urinate or defecate, and hot and cold flushes. The relative prominence of affective, cognitive and somatic features varies with type of disorder, between young people, and within the same young person over time.

Anxiety disorders may co-occur with each other and with other disorders such as depression, behaviour disorders and attention deficit disorder. There may be at least one common path in the aetiology of anxiety and behaviour problems in young people presenting with both. If no clear limits are set to expected behaviour then, as well as showing undesirable behaviour, the young person experiences a sense of potentially unlimited control, which is in itself anxiety-provoking. Instituting clear limits to behaviour, with predictable consequences if these are breached, not only results in a diminution of the undesirable behaviour, but can also lead to reduced anxiety without the need for a specific intervention. Each anxiety disorder has a different predominant age of onset, which implies a developmental influence on presentation.

Separation anxiety

- **Presentation**

This is the most common anxiety disorder, affecting 2–4 per cent of children. It most commonly presents in preschool or early school years and is characterised by repeated, unrealistic and preoccupying anxiety associated with actual or anticipated separation from a particular adult, usually a parent. The anxiety may result in difficulty settling at night, and reluctance to go to school or to be alone – this can be to the extreme of refusing to be alone in a room when others are in the house. Parents may report that the child follows them to the bathroom; younger children may physically cling to the parent. It may reach the point where the child is habitually allowed to sleep with the parents when this is not the cultural norm. The child may experience repeated intrusive nightmares, which in young children are usually non-specific, such as monsters. There may be associated cognitive and physical symptoms. The child may believe that harm will befall their parent or themselves if separated. The parent may also experience anxiety at the prospect of separation.

- **Assessment**

Assessment should explore the presenting features and likely precipitants. The child and the parents should ideally be interviewed, together and, if possible, separately. It may, however, have to be one of the aims of intervention to accomplish an individual interview with the child. The school may have additional information, even if the young person has not attended school for some time. The dynamics of the parent–child relationship need exploration, particularly the transmission of anxiety between them and to identify parental behaviours and anxieties that perpetuate the problem.

• Treatment

Treatment should consist of two strands, which may run simultaneously. One is specific treatment of the separation anxiety and the other is to address any presumed precipitants. These may include the birth of a sibling, a recent loss or threat of loss, illness in the family, and change of house or school. These issues should be addressed in further appointments and at home.

Specific interventions are mostly behavioural and usually involve graded exposure to separation starting in the situations defined by the family as least distressing.

Unintentional rewards for clingy behaviour should be identified and avoided. Separation should be rewarded with positive comment and praise, and the use of a star chart may be indicated. Cognitive treatment may be warranted, and can include identifying phrases that the young person may use for self-reassurance. Should parental expectations, anxiety or behaviour be a significant factor, then these should be addressed. There is insufficient evidence to support the use of medication. Outcome is usually good, with no evidence of continuity with adult disorders.

Phobic anxiety

• Presentation

Young people may develop specific phobias, often of particular objects, animals or situations. These can include spiders, dogs, blood, needles and heights. General phobias include being in a crowded place, going outside (as distinct from separation anxiety), and public performance. Phobias are present in 2–4 per cent of young people. Whilst girls and younger children report more fears, there are no clear gender or age patterns.

• Assessment

Assessment should include checking the range of situations to which the anxiety relates, the degree of anxiety experienced in the situation or in anticipation of it, and to what extent this impedes the young person's function. The important feature of phobic disorders is that the anxiety leads to habitual avoidance of the situation. This is because anxiety increases as the situation is anticipated and further as the situation/object is approached – the young person finds that their anxiety lessens on leaving the situation, which effectively rewards the young person for leaving it. Eventually, anxiety levels will increase sufficiently on anticipation of the object/situation that the young person will avoid it altogether.

• **Treatment**

Simple phobias are common and do not require treatment, providing they do not cause significant distress or dysfunction. The remainder are most successfully treated by graded exposure to the feared object. The principle here is that the young person becomes accustomed to situations that initially promoted moderate degrees of anxiety to the point that their discomfort is less and anxiety levels fall more quickly, thus making it easier to pass on to the next most anxiety-provoking situation from a hierarchy of situations drawn up by the child and parent.

The young person may be unable to complete this regime without assistance, and the most appropriate person to support the intervention should be identified. This may be the professional, a parent or someone else in whom the young person has confidence and who has the requisite support skills. Cognitive interventions may include identification of automatic negative thoughts pertaining to the object identified by the young person at times of exposure, and active selection of alternative (positive) thoughts. Younger children may also find selected phrases to assist self-reassurance helpful. Again, there is usually no indication to use medication, and outcome is normally good.

Social anxiety disorder

• **Presentation**

Although social anxiety disorder and social phobia are not technically the same, they greatly overlap with each other – and indeed with generalised anxiety disorder and with marked shyness. It is, however, important to exclude disorders in which young people may avoid or fail to seek social contact, such as pervasive developmental disorders. In social anxiety disorder there is a persistent fear of being with unfamiliar adults and peers in social situations, which may be expressed in the young person's behaviour: crying, tantrums or freezing. The young person may experience anxiety, fear or panic attacks in the situation, which are commonly accompanied by somatic symptoms. The disorder is present in about 1 per cent of the population, and more commonly presents in late childhood and early adolescence.

- **Assessment**

As well as a comprehensive assessment of the child, in social anxiety there is also a strong reliance on corroborative accounts as the young person may not be aware of the extent of their limitations.

- **Treatment**

Treatment should include an explanation of anxiety and its function, anxiety management and social skills training. Self-esteem work is also often undertaken. These treatments are most effectively delivered as group therapy, which has been shown to have positive effects that generalise beyond the group.

School refusal

School refusal may sometimes present during early adolescence, when it represents a combination of adolescent stress and the revival of an earlier overdependent parent–child relationship. The increased need for independence and autonomy posed by the demands of secondary school precipitates an avoidance of school. It is most common in early adolescence; however, it can occur at times of school transition with no gender differences.

- **Presentation**

The problem can manifest after a time of change at school or a period of illness. The unwillingness to go to school is often expressed openly and the young person may say there is a particular student or lesson that they dislike or find anxiety-provoking. Although not strictly defined as a mental health problem, it can be associated with anxiety symptoms or with associated physical complaints such as headaches or abdominal pain. The prompt exclusion of medical problems is essential in order to prevent the secondary elaboration of physical symptomatology. Delay in the recognition of the underlying psychological basis for the problem greatly exacerbates the difficulties.

• **Management**

School refusal is most appropriately managed by the education welfare service. There should be a clear and consistent approach to returning young people to school. The school should involve the parents, and if appropriate the child, in devising programmes or plans. Parents need to support the programme to introduce the young person back to school. They need to be firm about what is expected of the young person and resist the temptation to accede to the young person's distress. If there are concerns about parental commitment, this may be appropriately discussed with social services or addressed legally.

Sometimes it is helpful to devise a phased return into the school environment. There should be clear expectations for the child, and parents and teachers need to be consistent and firm in this. It is important to try to encourage the young person to return to school as soon as possible. The longer it is left, the more the young person will feel that getting back is insurmountable. The prognosis is not good for a significant minority of adolescents, up to one third failing to maintain regular school attendance. Follow-ups of young people into adult life have shown that they may have a predisposition to anxiety or agoraphobic symptoms (Berg *et al.* 1974). Where there have been long absences the school should involve the education welfare service and the education psychology service to advise on the process of reintegration. Tuition at home is usually an unhelpful strategy, as it can perpetuate the problem and impedes appropriate social and educational development. Cognitive-behavioural techniques can assist the young person to gain understanding of their difficulties and control over the situation. If there are concurrent problems with anxiety, they will need to be addressed using cognitive behaviour therapy and anxiety management. The role of the CAMHS is usually to manage severe anxiety or phobia associated with school refusal.

Generalised anxiety disorder

• **Presentation**

Young people experience generalised anxiety and tension that is not focused on one event or situation. This is often accompanied by somatic symptoms and non-specific complaints of ill health. Young people often seek reassurance and worry about their performance –

past, present and future. Most studies estimate prevalence at 3 per cent, but some as high as 6 per cent.

• **Assessment**

A comprehensive assessment as described above. A family history may be very significant and a family may describe itself as being 'worriers'.

• **Treatment**

Treatment includes anxiety management and cognitive therapy to address specific anxieties where present. If a family is made up of several people who worry, family therapy can be useful in helping them manage their anxieties rather than generate even more anxiety. However, many young people have continued symptoms on into adult life.

Case study: Tom

Tom is a 15-year-old boy with recurrent and intense fears of failure. This causes him to panic in situations requiring public performance, such as answering questions in class. He experiences gripping headaches in anticipation of situations where there is just the slightest chance of him being judged by others, and this has led to avoidance of these situations and resulted in poor school attendance.

Identify the likely distorted cognitions that Tom may have.

How would you help him to identify these?

Attachment disorders

Based on the work of Bowlby and Ainsworth already discussed in Chapter 6, it follows that if attachment with caregivers does not develop there might be sequelae. O'Connor and Zeanah (2003) argue that whilst there is a greater understanding of the needs of children who experience early deprivation, there is not an equal understanding about the nature of attachment related disturbances or strategies for intervention.

• **Presentation**

Broadly, there are two types of attachment disorder identified. The first is where children are indiscriminate about who they form 'attachment' to – they are inappropriately friendly with everyone and show little wariness. The second is where attachment is more defined in relation to the child's behaviour toward the caregiver. Children with insecure attachment, especially disorganised attachment, are at significant risk of later emotional and behavioural problems. Many children who do not form secure attachments may be children who are institutionalised or have a lack of consistent care (Allen 2007). However, attachment disorder may also be present when primary caregivers have a history of postnatal depression, unwanted pregnancy and/or other adverse perinatal events.

- **Assessment**

Assessment is often not comprehensively undertaken. O'Connor and Zeanah (2003) support the use of multiple methods of assessment, including comprehensive history of early childhood (which may often be lacking for children who have experienced early neglect and deprivation), history of concerning behaviours and observations. Questionnaires may also be useful but need to be used in conjunction with clinical history and observations. It is important that attachment disorder is not diagnosed without a clarity of context, as attachment is a two-way process. Children will show developmentally inappropriate social relationships and may also present as having an anxious relationship with caregivers and/or disinhibited behaviour (behavioural problems, inattention, poor concentration, aggression) or asocial behaviour (lack of empathy or ability to see another perspective) in which attention deficit hyperactivity disorder or autistic spectrum disorder may be mistakenly diagnosed. Learning disability may also need to be excluded as children who demonstrate friendliness to strangers may be doing so as they do not understand the contexts for different social relationships. O'Connor and Zeanah (2003) opine that the current DSM-IV and ICD criteria are inadequate for guiding clinical practice.

- **Treatment**

To date there is no known effective treatment for attachment disorders although several psychotherapeutic techniques are used based on very little evidence (Croft and Celano 2005). O'Connor and Zeanah (2003) are particularly critical of the dominance of holding therapy despite the lack of evidence. They argue that those that use it purport that it can facilitate attachment relationships, but that they have not examined the extent to which there is an improvement in the quality of attachment relationship (using reliable measures of attachment quality). Family therapy may be appropriate in some contexts but would be inappropriate if there is ongoing abuse (emotional or otherwise). Social cognitive treatment approaches may be more beneficial given that there is greater evidence of efficacy for changing specific behaviours (such as peer rejection).

From a front-line perspective, it is important that terms such as attachment disorder are not loosely used and there is awareness that other disorders need to be excluded before such a diagnosis should be made.

Panic disorder

Panic disorder is not commonly present in young people without other features of anxiety, and may accompany agoraphobia (fear of being in a place without immediate escape, e.g. outside the home, in a crowd). Indeed the current American classificatory system, DSM-IV-TR (American Psychiatric Association 2000), defines two panic disorders, one with and one without agoraphobia. A panic attack is a discrete, intense experience of fear or anxiety, with sudden onset, typically peaking at five to ten minutes and accompanied by several physical symptoms and cognitive features, particularly the fear held by the young person that he or she is going 'mad' or 'crazy'. Panic disorder is the recurrent, unexpected experience of panic attacks. Other possible causes of panic attacks, such as medical disorders and substance use, should be excluded. Panic attacks may occur in simple phobias or social anxiety.

Panic disorder most commonly presents in the mid- to late-teens and there is frequently a family history. Treatment, in addition to anxiety management and behavioural and cognitive therapy, may include tricyclic antidepressants or selective serotonin reuptake inhibitors, which 'block' panic attacks.

Obsessive–compulsive disorder

Counting rituals, magical thinking and repetitive touching occur normally in childhood, and obsessions (with idolised figures such as pop stars and with subjects or beliefs) are a part of normal socialisation in adolescence.

None of these show any relationship or continuity with obsessive-compulsive disorder (OCD).

Obsessions are recurrent, intrusive thoughts that are distressing and recognised by the young person as being their own thoughts (as distinguished from psychosis – described in Chapter 12) and not simply worries about everyday life. The young person may recognise them as thoughts that come into their head over and over again and will not go away. They often take up a significant amount of time and impair social and educational function. Unlike adults with the disorder, young people do not necessarily recognise that the content of the thoughts is excessive or irrational. Obsessions may also be in the form of images (e.g. a visual representation of an imagined road accident) and impulses that the young person has no conscious desire to act on (e.g. a strong urge to shout out obscenities in school assembly, or to break a valued object).

Compulsions are actions that the young person feels compelled to repeat usually in a very specific way in accordance with rules that the young person has generated to reduce distress that is usually associated with obsessions. These compulsive actions are either physical (typically hand-washing, arranging or checking objects) or mental (typically counting, repetition of words or phrases to oneself in a specific way). The young person (or parent) may recognise the problem as something that they have to do over and over again or that they have to do in a particular way, starting again if they do not get it right. By performing the compulsion the young person aims to prevent an imagined undesirable or traumatic event, which either has no bearing on the compulsive behaviour or is an extreme response to it. Again, unlike adult patients, the young person does not necessarily recognise the excessive or irrational nature of the behaviour.

A diagnosis of OCD can be made with the presence of either obsessions or compulsions. Young people with OCD usually present with a long history, not uncommonly dating to preschool years. The problem is usually identified because of their eventual inability to complete tasks at school or home, spending excessive time washing or dressing, and possibly engaging other family members in their rituals. Other causes of similar ritualistic behaviours and obsessions, such as occur in autism, schizophrenia and Tourette's syndrome need to be excluded. Depression and anxiety can also cause symptoms of OCD.

Treatment is more effective for compulsions than obsessions. The core component of intervention is 'response prevention': the young person draws up a hierarchy of compulsions and – starting with the least distressing – aims to stop the behavioural response. A greater degree of anxiety is experienced immediately on doing so, for which anxiety management and cognitive therapy may be helpful. The programme should be such that the anxiety is tolerable, and repeated blocking of the behavioural response will result in reduced experience of anxiety, allowing progress to the next most challenging behaviour in the hierarchy.

Complex or prolonged behaviours may be considered as a series of separate behaviours and broken down into their constituent parts, again addressing the least distressing component first. Medication has a role in many cases, and may even do so in children as young as six years. Long-term outcome is poorer than for other emotional disorders, particularly where there is a predominance of obsessions, and many young people continue to experience symptoms into adulthood.

Adjustment reaction

Adjustment reaction can be diagnosed when there is a significant emotional response to a stressful event. The symptoms abate within six months of onset. The event usually involves loss or harm, such as

---

Case study: Jodie

Jodie is eight years old. Her mother, Ms Mortimer, requests to see you in your role as the school nurse. Ms Mortimer tells you that she is concerned that Jodie is unhappy at school and not learning as well as she could because of this. She feels the schoolteachers are not concerned with Jodie's lack of progress. She would like you and the school to sort things out.

As the school nurse, what further information might you like?

It becomes clear that Jodie had been progressing well until four months ago when her schoolwork deteriorated a little. At school she is noted to be a little quieter but settles as the school day progresses. Ms Mortimer separated from Jodie's father about four months ago and Jodie has had no regular contact with her father since that time.

What would you do next?

---

bereavement, family separation, a serious accident or abuse. There is disagreement as to the maximum interval from the event to the onset of symptoms, which ranges from one month (ICD-10: WHO 1992) to three months (DSM-IV: APA 2000). The symptoms may include depression, anxiety and behavioural disturbance in any combination. If the diagnostic criteria are met for other disorders, such as those listed above or major mental disorders, then they 'trump' adjustment reaction.

Abnormal bereavement reaction

Abnormal bereavement reaction may be considered if there is a significant departure from the 'normal' sequence of grief, which is similar across age groups.

There are several stages of grief recognised in a 'normal' reaction to bereavement. Different authors describe these differently, with between three and six stages depending on what they include in each. There is an initial stage of shock, during which the young person may be in denial, numb and detached from events, and may direct much of their mental and physical activity towards the deceased person. Young people may talk about the deceased as if they were still alive, and act accordingly. This stage may last from several minutes to days, and can be returned to from later stages of grieving. Rituals associated with the death, such as formalised mourning and funerals are invariably found across cultures. These assist young people in moving on from this stage in particular.

Many Western societies have 'sanitised' death to the extent that young people may be deprived of this important aspect of socialised mourning. Common issues for families are whether to allow a child to see the dead body, and whether the child would understand what it is all about. There is evidence that young people have an understanding of the permanence of death from toddlerhood, and increasingly adopt cultural beliefs throughout childhood. One benefit of a child seeing the body, if they so choose, is that it enables them to say goodbye. It also prevents distressing elaborations of what the body might look like. Apart from most Western societies over the last 150 years, custom has been to involve young people in all aspects of bereavement.

In the next stage, the young person may express despair, anger, guilt, sadness, hopelessness, self-blame and worthlessness. There may be changes in behaviour, appetite and sleep. Children may have an egocentric view of the death, whereby they believe that something they did, or did not do (often unrelated or very remotely related), directly caused the death. This belief may persist, despite reassurance, for several years. Young people commonly have visual and auditory hallucinations of the deceased, which may be either comforting or distressing. Sometimes professional reassurance is needed that they are not going 'crazy'.

The final stage of adjustment, in which the young person takes on and enjoys usual activities with a reduction of the distressing emotions, may take several months or even years to achieve. At each stage there may be a return to aspects of previous stages, particularly at the anniversary of the death and other times such as birthdays and religious festivals. The content and duration of each stage varies considerably.

What discriminates between a 'normal' and 'abnormal' bereavement reaction is difficult to define, and it is not usually helpful to talk in these terms. Three features, however, can distinguish a significant departure from a normal reaction. First, the reaction may follow a normal course, but the young person experiences marked distress or greater than expected dysfunction, particularly slowing of physical and mental activity (psychomotor retardation). Second, one or more stages may be prolonged. For instance, there may be a marked or prolonged belief held by the young person that he or she is worthless or should have died too. Third, there may be additional features not normally found, such as distressing emotions, negative cognitions or hallucinations unrelated to the death.

The young person and their family may seek support in the form of simple counselling about the nature of grief and how best to manage. Assessment should include a full history of events about the death itself (the nature of the death, beliefs held by each family member about it, how the young person heard of the death), the family's response to the death (how the funeral was managed and who attended, how the family have grieved and how they tolerate each other's grieving) and any other changes in the family. Intervention should be directed to specific aspects of the grief that have not been achieved in addition to general education or counselling about the nature of grief.

Posttraumatic stress disorder

Posttraumatic stress disorder (PTSD) occurs in young people in response to experiencing or witnessing events that caused a threat of death or serious harm, such as a disaster, gross violence, traumatic accident, abuse, serious illness and medical procedures. To diagnose PTSD there must have been such an event and the response must persist for at least one month and involve at least one aspect of each of the following features:

- intense fear, helplessness, horror, disorganised or agitated behaviour

- repeated re-experience of the event through intrusive images, thoughts, repetitive play; or frightening dreams (which in young people may or may not be related to the event); or a reliving of the experience with hallucinations and flashbacks; or re-enactment of the event, particularly by young children; or intense distress at reminders of the event; or marked physiological arousal at reminders of the event

- persistent avoidance of things that may be associated with the event or which may be a reminder of it, such as places, objects, activities, people and conversations; or inability to recall important aspects of the event, feelings of detachment, restricted range of feelings, or sense of foreshortened future

- persistent symptoms of arousal, including poor sleep and concentration, irritability, exaggerated startle response and markedly increased vigilance.

Onset is defined as delayed if more than six months after the stressor, and the disorder is defined as chronic (or persisting) if symptoms last more than three months. Screening instruments have been developed but are not sensitive at detecting PTSD compared with screens for other disorders, particularly when completed by parents and teachers. Young people should be assessed individually, where possible, as well as in parent and family interviews. They are more likely than in other disorders to hide symptoms to protect friends or family members from their own suffering or out of feelings of loyalty to anyone implicated in a trauma.

Before specific interventions can be made, it is important to ensure the young person's general welfare, safety and protection. There may be issues to address within the family, particularly if the event was abuse, serious harm, or murder. The young person may be reassured at how common such symptoms are – generally found in about 30–40 per cent experiencing a natural disaster, higher than this in war, displacement and violence, and between 40 per cent and 50 per cent in repeated sexual abuse (Davis and Siegal 2000; Rodriguez, Vande Kemp and Foy 1998). Talking over the event may be helpful but premature counselling or formal debriefing may 'block' the natural resolution of symptoms. Sharing experiences with others who experienced the same or similar events in therapeutic groups may help the young person. Young people can be helped to understand the event further through play and verbal therapies. Behavioural and cognitive therapies can be helpful in managing anxiety and avoidance of specific places, and managing dreams, distressing emotions and intrusive thoughts.

References

Allen, J. (2007) 'Interventions for foster carers and adoptive parents of children who have experienced abuse and trauma.' In P. Vostanis (ed.) *Mental Health Interventions and Services for Vulnerable Children and Young People.* London: Jessica Kingsley Publishers.

American Psychiatric Association (2000) *Diagnostic and Statistical Manual of Mental Disorders* (4th edition). Text Revision (DSM-IV-TR). Arlington, VA: American Psychiatric Association.

Berg, I., Marks, I., McGuire, R. and Lipsedge, M. (1974) 'School phobia and agoraphobia.' *Psychological Medicine 4*, 428–434.

Croft, S. and Celano, M. (2005) 'Evaluating and managing attachment difficulties in children.' In S.S. Sexson (ed.) *Child and Adolescent Psychiatry* (2nd edition). Malden, MA: Blackwell Publishing.

Davis, L. and Siegel, L.J. (2000) 'Posttraumatic stress disorder in children and adolescents: A review and analysis.' *Clinical Child and Family Psychology Review 3*, 3, 135–154.

O'Connor, T. and Zeanah, C.H. (2003) 'Attachment disorders: Assessment strategies and treatment approaches.' *Attachment and Human Development 5*, 3, 223–244.

Rodriguez, N., Vande Kemp, H. and Foy, D.W. (1998) 'Posttraumatic stress disorder in survivors of childhood sexual and physical abuse: A critical review of the empirical research.' *Journal of Child Sexual Abuse 7*, 2, 17–45.

World Health Organization (1992) *The International Classification of Diseases, ICD-10 Classification of Mental and Behavioural Disorders.* Geneva: World Health Organization.

Further reading

Dwivedi, K.N. (2000) *Post-traumatic Stress Disorder in Children and Adolescents.* London: Whurr.

Flament, M.F. (1999) 'Obsessive-compulsive disorders.' In H-C. Steinhausen and F. Verhulst (eds) *Risks and Outcomes in Developmental Psychopathology.* Oxford: Oxford University Press.

Hill, P.D. (1994) 'Adjustment disorders.' In M. Rutter, E. Taylor and L. Hersov (eds) *Child and Adolescent Psychiatry: Modern Approaches* (3rd edition). Oxford: Blackwell Scientific.

Klein, R.G. (1994) 'Anxiety disorders.' In M. Rutter, E. Taylor and L. Hersov (eds) *Child and Adolescent Psychiatry: Modern Approaches* (3rd edition). Oxford: Blackwell Scientific.

Rapoport, J.L., Swedo, S. and Leonard, H. (1994) 'Obsessive-compulsive disorder.' In M. Rutter, E. Taylor and L. Hersov (eds) *Child and Adolescent Psychiatry: Modern Approaches* (3rd edition). Oxford: Blackwell Scientific.

Seligman, L.D. and Ollendick, T.H. (1999) 'Anxiety disorders.' In H-C. Steinhausen and F. Verhulst (eds) *Risks and Outcomes in Developmental Psychopathology.* Oxford: Oxford University Press.

Yule, W. (1994) 'Posttraumatic stress disorders.' In M. Rutter, E. Taylor and L. Hersov (eds) *Child and Adolescent Psychiatry: Modern Approaches* (3rd edition). Oxford: Blackwell Scientific.

CHAPTER 9

Behavioural Problems

This chapter has two parts. In the first we consider behavioural problems related to developmental aspects and in the second we focus on disorders which have a behavioural component to their presentation.

Behavioural problems related to development
Preschool children

Defiance, temper tantrums, impulsivity, breath holding, sleep problems and perceived lying are frequently noted around the ages of two to four years, when children need autonomy but do not have the skills for successful independence. Around 5 per cent of three-year-olds display severe tantrums (Richman, Stevenson and Graham 1982). Most of these behaviours are considered appropriate at certain developmental levels. They are often as a result of anger and frustration. Studies of US preschoolers show that around 8.3 per cent of children have behaviour difficulties at some point, with an excess of oppositional defiant disorders seen in this age group (Lavigne *et al.* 1993, 1996).

Temper tantrums, defiance, oppositionality, impulsivity
PRESENTATION

These behaviours are frequently shown by children of 18 months to 3 years. They often feel frustrated by conflicting desires to be, on the one hand, in control of their environment and, on the other hand, taken care of and pampered in a developmentally regressed way. Children of two to five years may show aggression in the form of temper tantrums, screaming, hurting others, or destroying toys or furniture. Aggressive behaviour is frequently a product of particular frustrations and a toddler's inability to manage them. It is usually directed toward parents during preschool years, and later towards siblings or peers. Verbal aggression increases between two and four years, and after three years revenge and retaliation can be prominent acts of aggression.

RISK FACTORS

When temper tantrums become overwhelming and persistent, there are often other contributing factors to continuing outbursts. These can be related to risk factors such as:

- family disruption
- inconsistent parental management
- witnessing of 'out-of-control' or aggressive behaviour in the family
- separation anxiety
- abuse
- developmental delay
- poor interpersonal relationships.

ASSESSMENT AND MANAGEMENT

When undertaking an assessment, as well as exploring parental expectation of behaviours for a given age, behaviours that parents are concerned about should be specifically clarified in detail. It is important to observe parental management of behaviours as part of the assessment, as that will prove useful in planning the management with the parents. Parental responses to the above behaviours determine the likelihood of the behaviours recurring and persisting. A parent who responds with punitive anger runs the risk of reinforcing the idea that emotionally 'out of control' responses are acceptable. Children can often be frightened by the strength and intensity of their own angry feelings, as well as those that they raise in their parents. Parents need to model and control their own anger and aggressive feelings, if they wish children to follow.

Most parents of children with such problems can become frustrated and horrified by their children's loss of control and displays of anger. Most problematic behaviour can be modified by consistent application of behavioural techniques discussed in Chapter 13.

Breath holding

Breath holding is very common during the first years of life. Infants and toddlers may frequently use it in an attempt to control their environment and their parents.

PRESENTATION

This behaviour can become problematic and concerning, as children may hold their breath until they lose consciousness. This can sometimes lead to seizures, which in turn lead to parental panic. However, there is no increased risk of later developing a seizure disorder in children.

MANAGEMENT

Parents are best advised to ignore the behaviour and leave the room in response. This eradicates most breath holding. This response should not be used if the child is physically unwell or has a respiratory problem. If breath holding continues and is coupled with other disruptive behaviours

---

Case study: Jacob

Ms Collins is a 21-year-old single mother. She has approached her health visitor for help. Her son Jacob, age three, has started to refuse to do anything she asks him. He often hits out when he has to do things that he does not like. She sends him to his room but he screams for hours and strips the wallpaper off the walls of his room. He has also started to use abusive language, but Ms Collins does not know why. He is fine at nursery and gets on well with other children. Ms Collins' partner left recently and Ms Collins is concerned that Jacob has heard arguments between her and his father. She feels that she is a useless mother. She no longer goes out with friends, as she is afraid that Jacob may treat a babysitter as he has treated her. She gives in to him a lot and feels he has now got the better of her; she is at the end of her tether and doesn't know what to do next. She feels there may be something wrong with him.

What should the health visitor do?

What would you do differently if Jacob's father were still part of the family?

---

and psychosocial factors then more intensive behavioural strategies may be necessary.

Lying and stealing

Lying can often be used by two- to four-year-olds as a way of playing with language, therefore it is important to keep it in perspective. Preschoolers learn cognitively and affectively by observing the reactions of parents. Lying is also a form of fantasy for young people, when describing the way they would wish things to be rather than how they are.

Before the age of five years, the concept of personal property is likely to be poorly developed. Therefore the concept of stealing in this age group cannot be meaningfully employed. From the age of six years onwards, stealing in its real sense can be possible. In the earlier age groups it can become confused with borrowing without permission. Children around the age of seven to nine years can become involved in stealing from shops or taking money from the home.

PRESENTATION AND MANAGEMENT

Regardless of age and development, intervention is warranted when lying becomes a frequent way of managing conflict and anxiety. Children should be given a clear message of what is acceptable. Sensitivity and support are important because children are developmentally vulnerable and therefore open to embarrassment and shame. When parents become unable to resolve or understand the situation then professional intervention is indicated.

Stealing can be impulsive, but the gratification derived does not satisfy underlying need. It can also be an expression of anger or revenge for real or imagined frustrations. In many instances children wish to be caught, it is one way for the child to manipulate and attempt to control interactions with parents. It is important to deal with an escalating problem as early as possible before the child raises the stakes and resorts to greater secrecy. Stealing can also be an indication of emotional or physical neglect.

Sleep problems and disorders

There are three distinct areas of sleep problems – difficulty in getting a child to go to bed, nightmares, and night terrors and sleepwalking, which together have rates of approximately 10 per cent in preschool children and 4 per cent in five to nine year olds (Richman 1981; Richman, Stevenson and Graham 1982). There can be different cultural and family expectations that determine whether problems with the onset of sleep are presented to professionals or not.

PRESENTATION AND MANAGEMENT
Nighttime sleeping
When there are problems with getting a child to bed, this is usually part of a wider picture, which includes defiance in several areas. The management is usually behavioural and the parents encouraged to parent with consistency and clarity.

Nightmares
These can occur at any age and may be associated with specific life events. Following trauma, they may occur in association with flashbacks and anxiety. A child who has experienced a nightmare is usually able to describe their nightmare to you. Their management involves identifying potential causes for the nightmares and addressing those issues. Recall of a nightmare may lead to some anxiety and the parents need to provide reassurance in a way that does not reinforce the anxiety.

Night terrors and sleepwalking
These are most common between the ages of six and nine years. Night terrors present with a history of the child often issuing a 'blood curdling' scream, sitting bolt upright while asleep, and appearing terrified. They may awake with no recall of what has just taken place. The child is not 'engageable', and appears disoriented and to be 'in a different world'. A child who has night terrors may also sleepwalk; these occur in the same stage of sleep. Most children outgrow night terrors and sleepwalking, and management largely comprises reassuring the parents, helping them ensure the child is safe if they sleepwalk. Parents also need to know that they should not try to wake the child during a night terror.

Eating problems in younger children
Problems encountered by preschool and younger children may range from being picky or faddy about food to severe problems such as non-organic

failure to thrive (when there is no identified medical cause to explain the reason that a child is failing to grow). It is unlikely that a child with a feeding problem other than the latter will become nutritionally deficient. Around 10 per cent of preschool children can show difficulties or problems with their feeding at some stage. However, the majority of these children will improve their eating habits as they get older, with no lasting consequences on their health (Butler and Golding 1986; Kedesdy and Budd 1998).

PRESENTATION
Feeding problems in early infancy (0–3 months)
Transient problems and minor setbacks in early feeding are common. Persistent and more severe problems are rare and require careful assessment. Some problems can be as a result of an underlying physical problem. However, if they are not, these difficulties may be a prelude to other behavioural problems.

Early eating or feeding problems include:

- rejection of the bottle or breast

- failure to suck

- crying – leading to difficulty in getting the child to feed

- diarrhoea

- colic

- constipation

- vomiting

- abdominal pain.

Rumination
Rumination can be defined as a repeated voluntary regurgitation of food, without associated nausea or gastrointestinal disorder, with a failure to gain weight. It usually occurs between the ages of 3 and 12 months and is possibly a reflection of the mother–child relationship. The relationship can be bound up with the symptoms in a complex interaction of cause and effect.

For the parent of a child who ruminates, their failure to feed the child successfully may render the act of feeding aversive. There is also a noxious odour of vomit, and clothes can become saturated. In severe cases treatment is urgent, as there are potential medical complications and the condition can become fatal.

Pica

Pica is the persistent ingestion of substances that have no nutritional value. Although onset is usually at 12–14 months, a diagnosis should not be made before the age of two years because infants often put objects in their mouths. Diagnosis is made if the behaviour occurs at least twice weekly and persists for more than one month.

Pica can be associated with psychiatric conditions such as autism, schizophrenia and Kleine–Levin syndrome. It is, however, more commonly associated with learning disability. Pica is important when recognising associated mental health issues such as autism. In children who do not have a learning disability it may also be a behavioural indicator of neglect or abuse. It can also be associated with poverty and parental mental illness.

Food avoidance emotional disorder

This disorder is restricted to early childhood. There is often a previous history of food restriction in the home and a presence of emotional disturbance such as phobias, obsessional behaviour, and refusal to attend school or depression. The avoidance is often of the same intensity as in older anorexic young people. However, distorted body image and fear of gaining weight are absent.

Pervasive refusal syndrome

The status of this as a syndrome is not yet determined and is controversial. This occurrence is rare and can be life-threatening. It consists of a profound and pervasive refusal to eat, drink, walk and talk. The child shows similar characteristics to anorexia, but rapidly manifests the other avoidant behaviours. The child may become totally regressive, and efforts to intervene may be met with terror or anger.

Childhood obesity

Childhood obesity is of concern primarily because of its persistence into later life. The psychological consequences are probably the most adverse effects of obesity. Children in nursery have already learned to associate obesity with a variety of less desirable traits, and obese children are the least popular in the peer group. Therefore obesity can result in low mood and poor self-esteem.

RISK FACTORS
The common risk factors for children developing more serious problems include:

- problems with social relationships

- adverse living conditions, such as overcrowding

- maternal mental health problems

- anxiety focused on the baby

- lack of social support.

MANAGEMENT OF EATING PROBLEMS IN PRESCHOOL OR YOUNGER CHILDREN
Children may be born prematurely or have physical problems at birth, which can make parents anxious, especially in relation to weight gain. Minor problems usually respond to providing parents with support and advice about feeding routines. Difficulties may arise from repeated battles at mealtimes, and children may miss stages in developing their own taste or in gaining a normal feeding routine. Behavioural techniques can be effective in establishing a normal eating pattern. Usually the less fuss made the better.

Disorders with a behavioural component on presentation
School-age children and adolescents
The problems presented here may be part of a broader problem which is presented through some of the behaviours discussed here.

Lying and stealing
Lying and stealing in isolation may be a problem in this age group. The presentation and management are not dissimilar to that in younger age groups, so a description is not repeated here. Generally, however, lying and

stealing tend to be part of a wider picture with other associated problems such as conduct disorder or family relationship difficulties.

Aggression

Aggression is probably one of the most concerning and distressing behaviours in this group of problems. Young people who are aggressive are often overly sensitive and may have a low threshold for perceiving and understanding aggression in others. They sometimes have poor social and problem-solving skills and tend to have automatic and impulsive responses. Often they will have difficulty in estimating the consequences of their behaviour and will use such behaviour to relate to their peer group. Intentional aggression may be primarily either a means to an end or to inflict physical or psychological pain. Hyperactive and clumsy children may be deemed aggressive due to accidental results of their behaviour. Aggression is often evidence of parental display of anger, aggression or punishment, which they may initiate when physically or psychologically hurt. Aggressive behaviour is also commonly associated with:

- conduct disorder
- attention deficit disorder
- specific learning disabilities (or difficulties)
- developmental delay.

RISK FACTORS

Aggression in childhood is also positively correlated to family un-employment, discord, criminality and mental health disorders (Farrington 2000; Stormont 1998). Factors that contribute to aggression include:

- gender – boys are reported more aggressive than girls, but aggression in girls is often less tolerated and more likely to be seen as abnormal or pathological
- size – large children are often more aggressive than smaller ones
- more active and impulsive children are perceived as more aggressive which in turn leads to them being more aggressive

- difficult temperament in infancy – has been shown to be related to later aggressiveness
- family size – children from larger families are often more aggressive than those from smaller families
- marital discord between parents and aggression in the home
- exposure to aggression in play and, controversially, on TV.

MANAGEMENT

The causes and motives of aggression should be identified. The management of aggression involves enabling young people to understand their problem. It includes the use of cognitive-behavioural techniques, which enable the young person to self-monitor their behaviour and to understand difficult situations. A method called self-instruction or self-talk (an internal dialogue which is used as a coping strategy to decrease the experience of anger arousal and to enhance the ability to manage an angry situation) is utilised to help them get through the difficulty. Usually the young person will benefit from learning problem-solving techniques and methods of relaxation.

The management plan within the home or school environment should focus on using a consistent approach, with defined boundaries and rules, which reward appropriate behaviour and encourage the young person's responsibility and autonomy.

Fire–related behaviour

Fire-related behaviour is on a continuum of severity from normal fire interest at one end of the spectrum to firesetting at the other. There are three sequential phases of fire behaviour: fire interest, fireplay and firesetting. Some children may never progress beyond the first level, whilst others may develop a career of risky and dangerous firesetting behaviour. The value of defining the level of fire-related behaviour is that it can help professionals to identify potential risk factors and the most appropriate care pathway.

PRESENTATION
Fire interest

Many children show what is considered to be a normal interest in fire at an early stage in their development. Studies of children aged five to nine years show that fire interest is almost universal. This includes: the desire to play with matches, interest in fire-related themes, making attempts to watch fires, and lighting matches or other combustibles. Children may express their curiosity in several ways, for example they may ask questions in relation to fire or they may incorporate fire scenarios into their play. Most children experiment with fire, and due to their inability to comprehend the inherent hazards of such an activity, experimentation can result in fire that is more serious than the child's level of risk would suggest. Interest should start to diminish around the age of nine or ten, beyond which this should no longer be considered as mere interest and requires investigation.

Fireplay

When fire interest extends to experimentation it becomes fireplay and is potentially serious, occurring mostly in boys between the ages of five and nine years. Fireplay may also include the collection of and experimentation with incendiary materials to see which are the most flammable or produce the most flamboyant effects. First-time fireplay seldom produces significant fire, however the probability for subsequent fireplay increases.

Firesetting

Children older than ten years should have learned the rules of fire safety and prevention. Should they continue with inappropriate behaviour beyond this point, with or without intervention, then they are deemed to show the risky and dangerous behaviour known as firesetting. The most concerning firesetting is when a child sets fires on their own, in an aggressive or angry manner or in an attempt to harm others.

RISK FACTORS

Young people may show a general pattern of behaviours – impulsive, overactive, mischievous, more prone to temper outbursts and destructive behaviour. Certain risk factors may also be present and these include:

- single-parent family

- absent father (e.g. working away from the family home)
- high level of marital discord
- overprotective parent who administers inappropriate harsh punishment
- parental mental illness
- domestic violence
- social isolation
- low self-esteem
- abuse
- early fire modelling within the family.

MANAGEMENT

Some local fire services run programmes for children and young people who start to show an interest in setting fires. It can be helpful for the child to be referred at an early stage. Whilst early fireplay can be addressed by the fire service, sustained firesetting requires specialist CAMHS intervention. In complex cases of firesetting it is important to have a multi-agency approach to managing the child's problems due to the potential danger to self and others.

Truancy

Truancy is defined as when young people stay off school without parental knowledge or permission or valid reason. It can start to become a problem for some young people during their secondary school years, usually during the final years of compulsory schooling, occurring more commonly in inner-city schools. Persistent truancy is unlikely in primary-school children.

Young people who truant often get ready for school, sometimes going in to register and then leaving the school premises. They commonly also exhibit other problem behaviours. Young people tend to truant in groups and will often say that they are bored with school. Those who spend their time alone are in a minority but are at greater risk of becoming involved in criminality. There is only a role for CAMHS when there is a clearly defined mental health disorder.

Conduct disorder

Nearly all young people at some time exhibit difficult or antisocial behaviour. Most have brief episodes of stealing or lying. Some may be involved in bullying or aggressive behaviour. The difference in a young person with conduct disorder is in the extent and severity to which difficult and antisocial behaviours are displayed and persist. However, there is considerable debate about whether this is a mental health disorder, although it appears in international classifications of diseases (Loeber *et al.* 2000). Up to 11 per cent of young people over ten years could be described as having a conduct disorder, depending on the defining criteria.

PRESENTATION

Conduct disorders are classified as either unsocialised or socialised. In unsocialised conduct disorder the young person usually presents with a pervasive difficulty in relating to their peer group, and in socialised conduct disorder they are usually well integrated with their peers. The diagnostic criteria include persistence of the behaviour difficulties for over six months and the presence of behaviours representing major violations of age-appropriate expectations, not just mischief or adolescent rebelliousness. Conduct disorder also often coexists with depression and/or substance misuse. Behaviours include:

- excessive levels of bullying or fighting
- severe destructiveness to property
- aggression
- stealing and repeated lying
- firesetting
- repeated truancy
- running away from home
- cruelty to other people and animals
- unusually frequent and severe temper tantrums
- defiant or provocative behaviour
- severe and persistent disobedience.

RISK FACTORS

In conduct disorders there is usually the coexistence of several of the following risk factors:

- socio-economically disadvantaged communities
- familial discord and large families
- poor parental child-rearing practices and modelling
- poor educational attainment or opportunities (especially specific reading disorder)
- genetic factors
- difficult temperament and personality
- poor physical health.

MANAGEMENT

Any form of treatment offered will depend on the motivation of the young person and the family; unfortunately this is often lacking. Cognitive-behavioural techniques can be helpful in a minority of cases, as can other forms of psychotherapy, such as behaviour and family therapy. Medication sometimes has a limited role to play in the treatment of conduct disorders, especially in those who have severe aggressive outbursts not associated

---

Case study: Jack

Jack is a seven-year-old boy who lives with his mother, younger sister and maternal grandmother, who dotes on him. He reminds his mother of his father, from whom she separated after he was convicted of violent assault; consequently she prefers the company of his younger sister. His mother brought Jack to see the GP because he frequently bites his sister at home and other children in the playground. Other parents have complained, and Jack is at risk of being expelled from school. During the interview she was angry with Jack and kept demanding to know why he continued to behave as he did despite her attempts to stop his bad behaviour. She has shouted at him, slapped and bitten him 'to show him what it's like' but his behaviour continues. However, on recounting an episode that she witnessed of him biting at school she smiled, and admitted that sometimes she finds it amusing and laughs at his behaviour. At this point Jack looked up at her and grinned.

What behavioural techniques has Jack's mother unwittingly used that have encouraged the biting?

How effective are the techniques that she has used to discourage the biting?

How should this be further assessed?

What is this assessment likely to demonstrate?

Outline an intervention to reduce the frequency of biting.

Does Jack's grandmother have a role to play, and if so what?

What advice should be given to the school?

---

with epilepsy, but this should only be given in consultation with specialist services. There has been recent discussion that parenting programmes based on social learning models are more effective than other types of parenting programmes (Scott 2008). However, much of this applies to those children under 12 years of age. Multisystemic Therapy (MST) offers promise for older children with conduct disorder but has yet to be used in non-specialist contexts (Scott 2008). The proactive nature of MST supports the engagement of unmotivated families.

References

Butler, M.R. and Golding, J. (eds) (1986) *From Birth to Five: A Study of Health and Behaviour in Britain's Five-year-olds.* London: Pergamon Press.

Farrington, D.P. (2000) 'Adolescent violence: Findings and implications from the Cambridge Study.' In G. Boswell (ed.) *Violent Children and Adolescents: Asking the Question Why.* London: Whurr Publishers.

Kedesdy, J.H. and Budd, K.S. (1998) *Childhood Feeding Disorders: Biobehavioural Assessment and Intervention.* Baltimore: Brooks Publishing Company.

Lavigne, J.V., Binns, H.J., Christofel, K.K., Rosenbaum, D., *et al.* (1993) 'Behavioural and emotional problems among pre-school children in paediatric primary care: Prevalence and pediatricians' recognition.' *Pediatrics 913*, 649–655.

Lavigne, J.V., Gibbons, R.D., Christofel, K.K., Arend, R. *et al.* (1996) 'Prevalence rates and correlates of psychiatric disorder among pre-school children.' *Journal of the American Academy of Child and Adolescent Psychiatry 35*, 2, 204–214.

Loeber, R., Burke, J.D., Lahey, B.B., Winters, A. and Zera, M. (2000) 'Oppositional defiant and conduct disorders: A review of the past 10 years, Part I.' *Journal of the American Academy of Children and Adolescent Psychiatry 39*, 12, 1468–1484.

Richman, N. (1981) 'A community survey of one to two-year-olds with sleep disturbances.' *Journal of the Academy of Child Psychiatry 20*, 281–291.

Richman, N., Stevenson J. and Graham, P. (1982) *Pre-school to School: A Behavioural Study.* London: Academic Press.

Scott, S. (2008) 'An update on interventions for conduct disorder.' *Advances in Psychiatric Treatment 14,* 61–70.

Stormont, M. (1998) 'Family Factors associated with externalising disorders in preschool children.' *Journal of Early Intervention 21,* 3, 232–251.

Further reading

Burke, J.D., Loeber, R. and Birmaher, B. (2002) 'Oppositional defiant disorder and conduct disorder: A review of the past 10 years, Part II.' *Journal of the American Academy of Child and Adolescent Psychiatry 41,* 11, 1275–1293.

Kazdin, A.E. (1997) 'Practitioner Review: Psychosocial treatments for conduct disorder.' *Journal of Child Psychology and Psychiatry 38,* 2, 161–178.

Neville, D., King, L. and Beak, D. (1995) *Promoting Positive Parenting.* Aldershot: Arena.

Neville, D., King, L. and Beak, D. (1995) *Promoting Positive Parenting of Teenagers.* Aldershot: Arena.

Sutton, C. (1999) *Helping Families with Troubled Children.* Chichester: Wiley.

Turk, J., Graham, P. and Verhulst, F. (2007) *Child and Adolescent Psychiatry: A Developmental Approach* (4th edition). Oxford: Oxford University Press.

CHAPTER 10

Neurodevelopmental Disorders

The term *Neurodevelopmental Disorders* encompasses a heterogeneous group of disorders of genetic, environmental, mixed or unsubstantiated aetiology that usually present in infancy or early childhood and have a chronic course, often into adulthood.

There are several dozen disorders included in this group, and this chapter will focus on two that are more likely to present with mental health problems. This is not to say that the other disorders, which present to mental health services less frequently, are any less deserving of consideration of their impact on the mental health of the individual.

Neurodevelopmental disorders may affect up to 3 per cent of the population and typically affect boys more frequently than girls. Interestingly for many neurodevelopmental disorders, the sex ratio approximates to 1:3.

These disorders can cause considerable health, social and economic problems, many of which are preventable or treatable. Their impact is experienced by the individual, the family, the community and society.

This chapter outlines the mental health aspects of attention deficit hyperactivity disorder (ADHD) and autism and related disorders.

Attention deficit hyperactivity disorder

The definition and classification of attention deficit hyperactivity disorder (ADHD) have changed significantly over the last two decades. The DSM and ICD classifications have come somewhat closer. ICD uses the terminology hyperkinetic disorder and DSM uses attention deficit hyperactivity disorder. The core features of ADHD comprise a triad of:

- inattention (decreased concentration and cognitive focus)
- hyperactivity (restlessness, overactivity relative to that required)
- impulsivity (lack of or significantly reduced forethought or consideration of consequences), which may be expressed verbally or behaviourally.

These cardinal features of ADHD are common characteristics of the behaviour of toddlers and preschool children. As the brain matures, so is the child able to restrict motoric behaviour, increase attention, and delay behavioural responses while consequences are considered. Hence, ADHD can be described as a neurodevelopmental disorder and presenting features should always be assessed relative to what would be expected for the individual's age. As in many other areas of development, this maturation is slower in boys than girls, and boys are at greater risk of developing the disorder.

Controversy endures about the definition of this disorder, diagnosis processes, and terms used to describe children with hyperactivity. There is also wide opinion on the aetiology and management of this disorder. There is debate about whether ADHD is a discrete diagnosis and whose interests are served in making the diagnosis and treating it using medication (Breggin and Breggin 1995). Professionals apply the diagnostic criteria with varying precision, and there is criticism that some apply the criteria too flexibly (Breggin and Breggin 1995). There may also be differences in the way professionals are trained to identify the disorder (Prendergast *et al.* 1988). The controversy is compounded by the amount of media attention this particular disorder receives. Sometimes parents and non-mental health professionals make an inaccurate diagnosis for themselves. This may lead to a lack of clear understanding among professionals and between professionals and families. The publication of practice guidelines (Pliszka 2007) goes some way to achieving a more consistent approach.

Differences in the definition of ADHD between countries and over time have resulted in wide variation (Green *et al.* 1999) in estimates of prevalence from as low as 1.3 per cent to 1.7 per cent in Europe (Gillberg, Carlstrom and Rasmussen 1983; Taylor *et al.* 1991) to 11 per cent or more in the US (Zametkin and Ernest 1999). Generally, community prevalent rates are estimated at around 4 or 5 per cent using DSM criteria, and around 2 per cent using the more stringent ICD criteria. ADHD has consistently been found to be approximately three times more common in boys than girls, with a peak in childhood, reducing in adolescence.

PRESENTATION

Inattention, overactivity, and impulsivity in excess of that seen in similarly-aged peers generally become apparent from mid-toddlerhood and later preschool years. These features may present in the following ways:

- Inattention
  - Poor concentration (manifested by significantly reduced ability to stay on task unprompted compared with peers).
  - Easily distracted (by extraneous stimuli and own thoughts).
  - Often shifts from one incomplete activity to another.
  - Recurrent difficulty in following instructions.
- Hyperactivity
  - Often physically overactive (relative to peers).
  - Often talks excessively.
  - Often finds it difficult to play quietly.
  - Often fidgets or squirms.
- Impulsivity
  - Often interrupts or intrudes on others (adults or peers).
  - Frequent difficulty turn taking (e.g. in games with other children, or blurting out answers to questions in class).
  - May engage in potentially hazardous activities without considering consequences (e.g. running across road, climbing out of windows).

Children may present to services with consequences of ADHD rather than its core features. A careful enquiry for features of ADHD should be made in any of the following presentations:

- Schools
  - Delayed educational attainment in the absence of a learning disability.

- ○ Disinterest in sustained academic activity.

- ○ Apparent forgetfulness or difficulty following instruction.

- ○ Poor relationships with peers (who are intolerant of the child's behaviour, particularly impulsivity).

- Social Services or social welfare non-governmental organisations

  - ○ Difficult-to-manage behaviour (that is impulsive or hyperactive).

  - ○ Increasingly harsh discipline used in ineffective attempts to manage these behaviours.

  - ○ Poor family relationships.

  - ○ Frequent apparent non-accidental injuries

- Youth Justice System (Police, Youth Courts, or Justice Social Workers)

  - ○ Recidivistic offending.

  - ○ Substance use.

RISK FACTORS

Several factors are implicated in the aetiology of ADHD or associated with it. These include:

- **Family history**

Biological parents of children with ADHD are more likely to exhibit ADHD or have a related disorder than are non-adoptive parents (van den Oord, Boomsma and Verhulst 1994).

Siblings of children with ADHD are two or three times more likely to have ADHD than are normal controls (Faraone and Biederman 1994).

- **Physical problems, particularly affecting the brain**

Cerebral palsy, epilepsy, and learning disabilities.

Prenatal exposure to alcohol, drugs and cigarettes.

25 per cent of children with traumatic brain injury have ADHD.

Lead or zinc poisoning.

- **Family factors**

Disruptions to early care giving (Jacobvitz and Sroufe 1987).

Parenting that is demanding, aversive and power assertive (Buhrmester *et al.* 1992).

Although diet is often cited by parents as having an influence, studies of this have been inconclusive. Most evidence arises from older studies with poor methodology. One recent study found generally increased levels of hyperactivity in preschool children as a result of eating food colouring and benzoate preservatives (Bateman *et al.* 2004). Children with pre-existing hyperactive behaviour were no more vulnerable to this effect.

ASSESSMENT

Assessment is multifaceted and should comprise multidisciplinary and ideally multi-agency input (Taylor *et al.* 2004). Assessment should be led by a trained specialist. It should comprise careful history taking that specifically identifies symptoms of inattention, impulsivity and hyperactivity. This history should be obtained from multiple informants who know the young person well, including caregivers/parents and teachers, and where feasible the child or young person themselves. This history may be supported by direct professional observations of the child at home and at school and by standardised rating scales completed by caregivers and teachers. Repeated use of the same scales at intervals is also useful in monitoring response to treatment. Sometimes psychometric assessments that directly test concentration and ability to control impulses can also be informative, though the diagnosis rests on careful elucidation of the history.

MANAGEMENT

Management of ADHD should also be multifaceted and is ideally delivered by the multidisciplinary team that has completed assessment (Taylor *et al.* 2004). Caregivers, teachers and any other adults directly involved with the young person should be provided with sufficient information (including written) about ADHD and its management in support of their interactions with the child. The family may be further supported by contact with support groups.

Although controversy still surrounds the use of psychostimulant medication in ADHD, this is one of the most highly researched areas. More recent studies have been larger with more robust designs and have reconfirmed that medication is more effective on the core symptoms of ADHD than psychosocial treatment alone (Jensen *et al.* 1999). Medication is a recommended first-line intervention followed by psychosocial intervention, which may be required in the treatment of co-existing disorders.

The most commonly prescribed psychostimulant is methylphenidate which comes under a variety of names in a variety of formulations. However, up to 30 per cent of children with ADHD show no or minimal response to psychostimulant medication. Effectiveness may be limited by unwanted side effects, which can include decreased appetite with weight loss, agitation, nausea, abdominal pain, tics, palpitations, headache, dizziness and increased blood pressure. Second line treatments include atomoxetine and clonidine. There is no evidence to support the use of so-called 'drug holidays' for avoiding long-term effects. However, monitored periods off medication are valuable at intervals across adolescence in determining continued effectiveness and, therefore, need for medication, and some families prefer to stop medication over school holiday periods. Although there are concerns that psychostimulants are a drug of abuse, their use in ADHD reduces the risk of onset of substance use disorders in adolescence by 50 per cent (Faraone and Wilens 2003).

There may be subgroups of children with ADHD who particularly benefit from psychosocial intervention (Swanson *et al.* 2002), which may influence long-term outcome (Swanson *et al.* 2001). Effective psychosocial interventions include parent training (Sonuga-Barke *et al.* 2001) and strategies for reducing adult demands and intrusion (Morrell and Murray 2003). Although parent involvement has a low impact on ADHD symptoms, it can have a significant impact on internalising symptoms and academic problems (Corcoran and Dattalo 2006).

Studies of diet and dietary supplement including omega-3 fish oils have shown uncertain benefit (Clayton, Hanstock and Garg 2007).

Strategies to support the child in the classroom should be based on specialist assessment, taking account of teacher and teacher aide reports and direct observation. They should be tailored to the individual child and may include:

- the use of clear simple statements

- breaking down multi-task instructions

- ensuring that the child understands what they are required to do

- arranging the classroom so that the child sits away from extraneous distractions

- breaking activities down to shorter time periods with frequent timed breaks (e.g. 'ten minutes on, ten minutes off' in younger children).

These strategies can enhance the likelihood of success of reducing disruptive behaviour and improving on-task behaviour (Miranda, Jarque and Tárraga 2006), which should be rewarded as frequently as possible. A detailed Educational Psychology assessment is invaluable where there have been significant problems in school.

There is some evidence to support the effectiveness of self-regulation interventions (self-monitoring with reinforcement, self-management and self-reinforcement) in children with ADHD (Reid, Trout and Schartz 2005).

Case Study: Oliver

Oliver is a six-year-old boy who is frequently teased by his peers and acts like the 'clown of the class'. He often blurts out in class, runs around, fails to complete tasks set in class, is unable to sit still during 'quiet time', and in the playground has been observed to disrupt other children's games, much to their chagrin. His teacher has discussed this with his parents, who have described Oliver's behaviour at home as stressful; they don't feel able to have family days out because he often runs off. And yet, he becomes more disruptive when they try to keep him indoors for his own safety.

If you were Oliver's teacher, how might you approach this with the parents? Who else might you discuss this with?

What would be the most appropriate service to refer Oliver to? And who might be best placed to make this referral?

How might you be involved in Oliver's ongoing management?

Autism and related disorders

This is a group of disorders around which there is considerable controversy and misunderstanding (Wing 1996). These disorders are not common although their impact can be considerable. Two (not necessarily contrary) ways of considering autism and related disorders are: to view them on a broad spectrum from 'no disorder' through to core autism; and to view them as discrete disorders. Terminology for the group includes *Autism Spectrum Disorders (ASD)* and *Pervasive Developmental Disorders (PDD)*.

CHARACTERISTICS AND PRESENTATION OF AUTISM

Autism is characterised by a triad of features that affect function in all situations (see Table 10.1):

- impairment of social interactions (with impaired ability to understand social behaviour and contexts)

- impairment of reciprocal communication (with impaired ability to understand and use verbal and non-verbal communication)

- restricted, repetitive repertoire of interests/activities particular to that child (with impaired ability to think and behave flexibly).

There is usually:

- an abnormal development from infancy, though often these features may not be recognised at the time

- a history manifesting in preschool years, though may not present to services until later years.

There may additionally be cognitive impairment.

There is evidence that the prevalence of autism (and related disorders) has increased since the late 1980s (Fombonne 1999), though it is unclear whether this reflects an increased incidence in the population rather than a broadening of the definition or improved detection. Recent studies estimate the prevalence of autism at 6–9 per 10,000 individuals. The condition is three to four times more common in boys.

In addition to the core features, young people with autism may also present with associated (i.e. not diagnostic) features, which include fears, phobias, sleeping and eating disturbances, tantrums, aggression, self-injury and abnormal sensory response, such as intolerance of noise,

Table 10.1 Core triad of symptoms of autism		
Impairment of reciprocal social interactions	Impairment of reciprocal communication	Abnormal repertoire of interests or activities
• Inadequate appreciation of socio-emotional cues • Poor use of social signals • Lack of social or emotional reciprocity • Lack of emotional response to others • Failure to form developmentally-appropriate peer relationships • Lack of spontaneous sharing of interests, achievements, or enjoyment	• Delayed development or lack of language • If language is present, lack of social use of language (verbal and non-verbal) • Poor flexibility in expression (repetitive use of idiosyncratic language) • Poor variation in cadence and gesture • Impairment of imaginative play	• Adherence to rigid routine in daily activities • Preoccupation with unusual objects or parts of objects • Non-functional rituals or routines • Preoccupation with unusual interests and non-functional aspects of objects • Resistance to change • Repetitive stereotyped mannerisms (e.g. hand flapping)

preoccupation with texture, high sensitivity to taste, high pain threshold and preoccupied self-stimulation, such as spinning self (balance) or spinning objects (visual).

ASSESSMENT AND DIAGNOSIS OF AUTISM

Assessment should comprise a full history from informants (caregivers, preschool teachers). Standardised rating scales and semi-structured interviews can assist in accurately identifying symptoms and assessing functional ability.

Diagnosis requires qualitative impairment of functioning in all three areas of the triad of developmental abnormalities with onset (though not necessarily presentation) before the age of three years.

Early detection is important: there is evidence that earlier interventions lead to better functionality in later life (National Research Council 2001). Thus, primary care workers and preschool teachers can promote better outcomes through early detection by having a 'high index of suspicion' if parents report that 'something is odd or different' about their infant. Early features that distinguish infants who later receive a diagnosis of autism are (Baranek 1999; Werner *et al.* 2000):

- repeated failure to respond to their name being called

- sustained failure to distinguish a parent's voice (and parents frequently calling the infant's name)

- reduction in use of language (including preverbal language) after one year

- having an unusual response to at least one of the senses.

CAUSES OF AUTISM

Autism (and related disorders) has a greater genetic basis compared with other mental health disorders in childhood (Rutter 2000). There are many studies that support this. Siblings of a child with autism have substantially higher rates of the disorder than the general population (2–6%). It is likely that there are multiple interacting genes involved on more than one chromosome.

Autism is also associated with the presence of medical disorders. One study was erroneously reported to have found an association between the MMR (measles, mumps and rubella) vaccine and autism. Further study has not supported this link. However, the MMR vaccine is given around the time of onset of symptoms and it is a question parents may raise. Neither is there evidence to support the earlier theories held mid last century of 're-frigerator parents', whose supposed emotional frigidity induced autism in their children.

Other disorders on the autism spectrum

- **Atypical autism** is similar to autism but not all diagnostic criteria are fulfilled, or onset may be after three years of age.

- **Asperger syndrome** is characterised by impairment of social interaction and an abnormal repertoire of interests and activities, as in autism. There is no delay in cognitive development or the development of speech and language (though use of language may appear odd, being over-formal or stilted).

- **Childhood disintegrative disorder** presents with normal development in the first two years of life and marked sustained regression with an onset after toddlerhood and before the age of ten years. There is progressive loss of language, behavioural changes, incoordination, and loss of bowel or bladder control.

- **Rett's syndrome** is the most discrete PDD. It has an onset following normal development at 7–24 months and presents in girls only with impairment of speech and hand skills, with hand wringing and other midline hand movements, and loss of purposeful movement. Social development stops in toddlerhood. The cause of Rett's syndrome is unknown.

MANAGEMENT

There is an array of effective interventions available to assist in the management of autism spectrum disorders. The specific treatments selected should be tailored to the individual child and based on a detailed assessment of need. Needs may change over time and with circumstance, and they will depend on the child's developmental attainment. There are also many unproven 'cures' that are periodically touted: caution must be exercised when claims are made, particularly about amelioration of core features of autism, often based on one poorly-designed study. Effective interventions include:

- **Education** – teaching the child specific skills and behaviour is the most beneficial and potent intervention (National Research Council 2001). This is usually highly intensive, repetitive work, delivered individually or in a small group setting. Examples include:

    ○ **Contemporary Applied Behaviour Analysis** (ABA; which incorporates language, developmental and milieu approaches into a behavioural framework)

    ○ **Developmental-Social Pragmatic** (which utilises cognitive and socio-cultural approaches).

    Whilst each school for children with autism may have its own 'package' of programmes, these should be delivered flexibly to meet the individual child's needs.

- **Family and parent/caregiver support and advocacy** – the provision of information about the disorder, its management, and resources available locally improves outcome (Whitaker 2002). Parents may need support in acceptance of their child having the disorder, support in the management of behaviour, and financial support or advice. Parent-run support groups are increasingly available and able to meet these needs.

- **Specific individual therapies** – the child or adolescent with autism may benefit from a therapy directed at a particular need: physiotherapy, occupational therapy, speech and language therapy, behaviour therapy, and, in some older adolescents, industrial or vocational therapy aimed at achieving optimal gainful employment.

MEDICATION

Whilst there is no psychopharmacological 'treatment' of autism, some autistic features that pose significant risk or dysfunction in the individual warrant a trial of medication as an adjunct to behaviour therapy. Antipsychotic medication can be used in the management of aggressive, self-injurious and repetitive behaviours; SSRIs in anxiety, obsessions, and repetitive behaviours; and clonidine (and to a lesser extent stimulant medication) might be of benefit in overactivity. Benefit from medication is often limited by side effects, which is an indication for starting at a low dose and increasing slowly. Medication is considered after a failed or partial response to behavioural intervention, environmental modification, and provision of respite, though it may be used sooner in serious repetitive self-injurious behaviour. Co-existing disorders should receive appropriate treatment.

Case Study: Peter

Peter is nearly three years old and his parents have been concerned for some time that he is not as engaged with them as they would have hoped. They are unable to identify a particular time from when this first became apparent. He used to call out 'Dada' and 'Mama' during parent–child interactions, but this has stopped. He seems to be more interested in the flickers made by shadows moving behind his bedroom blinds than he is in his toys. And if he were to pick up a toy car, for instance, he doesn't play with it as they might have expected him to; instead he'll spend seemingly inordinate periods of time fascinated by spinning the wheels on it. They were particularly upset when the parents of another child at a recent three-year birthday party made a disparaging remark about Peter after he had shown no interest in playing with the others there.

Peter's parents decide to chat about him with the nurse at their local Health Centre. What should the nurse advise them?

What form of assessment should be planned and what investigations undertaken?

What is the most likely diagnosis? A comprehensive assessment might take several months and indeed some aspects of the developmental assessment would necessarily be postponed. What could be achieved in the interim?

References

Baranek, G.T. (1999) 'Autism during infancy: A retrospective video analysis of sensorimotor and social behaviours at 9–12 months of age.' *Journal of Autism and Developmental Disorders* 29, 213–224.

Bateman, B., Warner, J.O., Hutchinson, E., Dean, T. *et al.* (2004) 'The effects of a double-blind, placebo-controlled artificial food colouring and benzoate preservative challenge on hyperactivity in a general population sample of school children.' *Archives of Diseases in Childhood 89*, 506–511.

Breggin, P. and Breggin, G.R. (1995) 'The hazards of treating "Attention-Deficit/Hyperactivity Disorder" with methylphenidate (Ritalin).' *Journal of College Student Psychotherapy 10*, 2, 55–72.

Buhrmester, D., Whalen, C.K., Henker, B., MacDonald, V. and Hinshaw, S.P. (1992) 'Prosocial behaviour in hyperactive boys: Effects of stimulant medication and comparison with normal boys.' *Journal of Abnormal Child Psychology 20*, 103–121.

Clayton, E.H., Hanstock, T.L. and Garg, M.L. (2007) 'Long chain omega-3 polyunsaturated fatty acids in the treatment of psychiatric illnesses in children and adolescents.' *Neuropsychiatrica 19*, 2, 92–103.

Corcoran, J. and Dattalo, P. (2006) 'Parent involvement in treatment for ADHD: A meta-analysis of the published studies.' *Research on Social Work Practice 16*, 6, 561–570.

Faraone, S.V. and Biederman, J. (1994) 'Is attention deficit hyperactivity disorder familial?' *Harvard Review of Psychiatry 1*, 271–287.

Faraone, S.V. and Wilens, T. (2003) 'Does stimulant treatment lead to substance use disorders?' *Journal of Clinical Psychiatry 64*, Supp 11, 9–13.

Fombonne, E. (1999) 'The epidemiology of autism: A review.' *Psychological Medicine 29*, 769–782.

Gillberg, C., Carlstrom, G. and Rasmussen, P. (1983) 'Hyperkinetic disorders in children with perceptual, motor and attentional deficits.' *Journal of Child Psychology and Psychiatry 24*, 233–246.

Green, M., Wong, M., Atkins, D., Taylor, J. and Feinleib, M. (1999) *Diagnosis of Attention-Deficit/Hyperactivity Disorder.* Technical Review no. 3 (Prepared by Technical Resources International, Inc.) AHCPR Publication no. 99–0050. Rockville, MD: Agency for Health Care Policy and Research.

Jacobvitz, D. and Sroufe, L.A. (1987) 'The early caregiver–child relationship and attention-deficit disorder with hyperactivity in kindergarten: A prospective study.' *Child Development 58*, 1496–1504.

Jensen, P.S., Arnold, L.E., Richter, J.E., Severe, J.B. *et al.* (1999) 'Moderators and mediators of treatment response for children with attention-deficit/hyperactivity disorder – The multi-modal treatment study of children with attention-deficit/hyperactivity disorder.' *Archives of General Psychiatry 56*, 1088–1096.

Miranda, A., Jarque, S. and Tárraga, R. (2006) 'Interventions in school settings for students with ADHD.' *Exceptionality 14*, 1, 35–52.

Morrell, J. and Murray, L. (2003) 'Parenting and the development of conduct disorder and hyperactive symptoms in childhood: A prospective longitudinal study from 2 months to 8 years.' *Journal of Child Psychology and Psychiatry 44*, 4, 489–508.

National Research Council (2001) *Educating Children with Autism.* Washington, DC: National Academy Press.

Pliszka, S. (2007) 'Practice Parameters for the assessment and treatment of children and adolescents with attention deficit hyperactivity disorder.' *Journal of the American Academy of Child and Adolescent Psychiatry 46*, 894–921.

Prendergast, M., Taylor, E., Rapoport, J.L., Bartko, J. *et al.* (1988) 'The diagnosis of childhood hyperactivity: A US–UK cross-national study of DSM-III and ICD-9.' *Journal of Child Psychology and Psychiatry 29*, 3, 289–300.

Reid, R., Trout, A.L. and Schartz, M. (2005) 'Self-regulation interventions for children with attention deficit/hyperactivity disorder.' *Exceptional Children 71*, 4, 361–377.

Rutter, M. (2000) 'The genetic studies of autism: From the mid-1970s into the millennium.' *Journal of Abnormal Child Psychology 28*, 3–14.

Sonuga-Barke, E.J.S., Daley, D., Thompson, M., Laver-Bradbury, C. and Weeks, A. (2001) 'Parent-based therapies for preschool attention-deficit/hyperactivity disorder: A randomized, controlled trial with a community sample.' *Journal of the American Academy of Child and Adolescent Psychiatry 40*, 4, 402–408.

Swanson, J.M., Kraemer, H.C., Hinshaw, S.P., Conners, C.K. *et al.* (2001) 'Clinical relevance of the primary findings of the MTA: Success rates based on severity of ADHD and ODD symptoms at the end of treatment.' *Journal of the American Academy of Child and Adolescent Psychiatry 40*, 168–179.

Swanson, J.M., Arnold, L.E., Vitiello, B., Abikoff, H.B. *et al.* (2002) 'Response to commentary on the multimodal treatment study of ADHD (MTA): Mining the meaning of MTA.' *Journal of Abnormal Child Psychology 40*, 168–179.

Taylor, E., Döpfner, M., Sergeant, J., Asherson, P. *et al.* (2004) 'European clinical guidelines for hyperkinetic disorder – first upgrade.' *European Child and Adolescent Psychiatry, 13*, Supplement 1, 7–30.

Taylor, E.A., Sandberg, S., Thorley, G. and Giles, S. (1991) *The Epidemiology of Childhood Hyperactivity.* London: Oxford University Press.

van den Oord, E.J., Boomsma, D.I. and Verhulst, F.C. (1994) 'A study of problem behaviours in 10–15 year old biologically related and unrelated international adoptees.' *Behaviour Genetics 24*, 193–205.

Werner, E., Dawson, G., Osterling, J. and Dinno, N. (2000) 'Brief report: Recognition of autism spectrum disorder before one year of age – A retrospective study based on home videotapes.' *Journal of Autism and Developmental Disorders 30*, 157–162.

Whitaker, P. (2002) 'Supporting families of preschool children with autism.' *Autism 6*, 4, 411–426.

Wing, L. (1996) *The Autistic Spectrum: A Guide for Parents and Professionals.* London: Constable and Robinson.

Zametkin, A.J. and Ernest, M. (1999) 'Current concept problems in the management of attention deficit hyperactivity disorder.' *New England Journal of Medicine 340,* 1, 40–46.

Further reading

Attwood, T. (2007) *The Complete Guide to Asperger's Syndrome.* London: Jessica Kingsley Publishers.

Frith, U. (2003) *Autism: Explaining the Enigma* (2nd edition). Oxford: Blackwell.

Gillberg, C. (1995) *Clinical Child Neuropsychiatry.* Cambridge: Cambridge University Press.

Munden, A. and Arcelus, J. (1999) *The ADHD Handbook: A Guide for Parents and Professionals.* London: Jessica Kingsley Publishers.

Volkmar, F.R. (ed.) (2007) *Autism and Pervasive Developmental Disorders* (2nd Edition). Cambridge University Press.

Websites

www.autism.org (Autism Collaboration)

www.nas.org.uk (National Autistic Society)

CHAPTER 11

Self-harm

Self-harm is a term that covers a variety of behaviours, with a multitude of different functions and a wide range of intentions. Self-harm in adolescence is common, whereas completed suicide is relatively uncommon, especially in those under 16 years of age. The terms deliberate self-harm (dsh) and suicide/parasuicide are falling out of fashion. The first is often felt to be pejorative and implies blame, which can be unhelpful. The second term is misleading as most people who self-harm do not want to kill themselves. In the UK, young people account for around 5 per cent of non-accidental self-harm episodes referred to hospital (Hawton, Fagg and Simkin 1996). Some 7–14 per cent of adolescents will self-harm at some time in their life, and 20–45 per cent of older adolescents report having suicidal thoughts at some time (Hawton and James 2005). Many attempts of self-harm remain hidden and therefore accurate prevalence figures are difficult to establish. Hawton *et al.* (2002) found that 6.9 per cent of a school population of 15 and 16-year-olds had engaged in an act of deliberate self-harm in the previous year. Only 12.6 per cent of these episodes had led to a hospital visit. These figures are comparable with US data (Centers for Disease Control 1990). As many as 30 per cent of adolescents who self-harm report previous episodes, many of which have not come to medical attention. At least 10 per cent repeat self-harm during the following year, with repeats being especially likely in the first two or three months (Hawton and James 2005). More recently self-harm appears to be increasing and in some circles is seen as an appropriate response to stress. Sometimes groups of young people self-harm together and having a friend who self-harms may increase a young person's chances of doing it as well. Suicidal ideation is relatively common among adolescents;

precipitating events may be non-specific; acts of self-harm are often impulsive; and secrecy and denial are common making prevention more difficult. Self-harm is not usually a disorder in itself, but indicative of other problems which may or may not be related to mental health.

PRESENTATION

Self-harm may present directly by:

- an overdose (the usual method of deliberate self-harm, analgesics being most commonly used)
- scratching or cutting the skin
- self-burning
- banging the head and/or self-punching
- self-strangulation
- hair pulling
- becoming involved in risky or dangerous behaviour (such as involvement in joy-riding, substance use, criminal activity)
- dangerous or unwanted sexual relations.

Other features may include:

- stated intent to self-harm
- evidence of ideas or plans about self-harm (e.g. school essays, shared diary)
- using self-harm as a means of dealing with feelings, as it often provides a release from difficult thoughts
- acute distress
- hostility and lack of communication
- poor skills in dealing with problems (especially social problems)
- a sense that self-harm brings about a degree of control for the young person.

Sometimes self-harming may be seen as a 'cry for help'. But it is essential not to dismiss a young person's distress, as they may be dealing with some difficult feelings, such as depression, anxiety, anger, grief or hopelessness, and presentation may be related directly to the escalation or arrival of a social problem (such as bullying, family discord).

RISK FACTORS

Factors associated with self-harm include:

- previous self-harm
- substance use
- presence of a mental health problem such as depression
- being in a vulnerable high-risk group
- experienced physical, emotional or sexual abuse
- being lesbian, gay or bisexual
- loss of relationship
- poor or inadequate coping skills
- family history of self-harm and suicidal behaviour
- availability of means (availability of firearms increases likelihood of completed suicide)
- family discord
- parental mental illness and/or parental substance use
- intercultural stressors, especially for South Asian females
- school and peer problems
- unemployment
- poverty/homelessness.

Young people who self-harm typically exhibit:

- negative feelings and traits
- feelings of insufficiency and low self-esteem
- distrust of others
- lack of control
- lack of supportive relationships and low family cohesion
- cognitive distortions and attribution styles

- responses to problems using maladaptive cognitive strategies relating to expectancies, commitments and explanations for events.

The physical severity of the self-harm is not a good indicator of suicidal intent because adolescents are often unaware of the relative toxicity of substances such as paracetamol, which people may incorrectly assume to be harmless. Many episodes of self-harm are impulsive and not repeated. It can be difficult for families and professionals to understand why young people self-harm. Self-harm for some is a strategy for coping with acute distress. It can also be a form of self-punishment. Young people can perceive deliberate self-harm as an effective method of ensuring they are heard. It is important to try and listen without being judgemental or critical. It is also important not to panic. Unless you have the necessary skills, it is probably more appropriate to refer to someone who is able to assess and manage risk. It may be useful to help the young person think about self-harm as a problem that needs to be sorted. It is also important not to promise that the self-harm will not be disclosed as this may become necessary if there is increased risk.

A further concern is that self-harm is a risk factor for completed suicide, or can result in unintended serious injury or fatality. Among adolescents who harm themselves, the factors that are most likely to be associated with a higher risk of later suicide include:

- male gender
- older age
- social isolation
- high suicidal intent (e.g. using dangerous and/or violent method)
- psychosis
- depression
- feelings of hopelessness.

The risk of suicide after deliberate self-harm lies between 0.24 per cent and 4.30 per cent (depending on the population and type of study). Psychological postmortem studies of suicides show that a psychiatric disorder (usually depression, rarely psychosis) is present at the time of death in most adolescents who die by suicide. A history of behavioural disturbance, substance misuse, and family, social and psychological problems is common. There are strong links between suicide and previous self-harm: between a quarter and a half of those committing suicide have previously carried out a non-fatal act (Hawton and James 2005). It can be difficult to identify young people at risk of self-harm, even though many older adolescents who are at risk consult their general practitioners before they self-harm.

ASSESSMENT

The National Institute for Clinical Excellence (NICE) and the National Collaborating Centre for Mental Health (NCCMH) have published a guideline for the NHS in England and Wales on the care of people who self-harm. The guideline makes recommendations for the physical, psychological and social assessment and treatment by primary and secondary services of people in the first 48 hours after an episode of self-harm. It covers acts of self-harm that are an expression of personal distress and where the person directly intends to injure him/herself, for example through cutting or poisoning (overdosing) (NICE 2004). Following a serious self-harm episode, attendance at an accident and emergency department should be considered to ensure that any immediate medical concerns are addressed. All events of self-harm should be taken seriously, even if they seem to be superficial, although superficial cutting rarely requires immediate medical attention. There needs to be a risk assessment and the development of a management plan. There needs to be clarification of whether the episode was impulsive or planned, whether a note was left, whether alcohol or other drugs were also ingested, what the young person expected might happen, how the young person feels about the overdose, what supports are in place for the young person, and what is likely to prevent the young person repeating the attempt. The guidelines recommend paying special attention to: confidentiality, young person's consent (including Gillick competence), parental consent, child protection issues and use of the Mental Health Act and the Children Act.

MANAGEMENT

Admission to a medical ward of any young person who has self-harmed is recommended (NICE 2004) and they should be assessed by a specialist the next day. All young people who have deliberately self-harmed should as a minimum be discussed with a child and adolescent psychiatrist or specialist nurse. Treatment goals, depending on need, can include:

- treat associated mental illness
- prevent future self-harm
- improve coping skills
- reduce distress
- prevent suicide
- extend the time between self-harm
- reduce injury severity.

(Royal Australian and New Zealand College of Psychiatrists 2005, p.7)

If the self-harm has occurred in the context of a disorder such as depression, poor self-esteem, poor social skills, those issues will need to be addressed. For all children and young people, caregivers should be advised to remove all means of self-harm as is practicable, including medication, before the child or young person goes home as a means of reducing further risk.

For those young people who do not have a mental health problem, there may still be benefits in exploring more appropriate coping strategies with them. Cognitive behaviour therapy (CBT), problem solving therapy (PST), dialectical behaviour therapy (DBT) and interpersonal therapy (IPT) are all forms of psychological treatment with proven effectiveness for helping people with depression, anxiety disorders and other mental health problems. There are no physical side effects to these therapies. There is relatively good evidence for the effectiveness of DBT (Linehan 1993), which acknowledges the importance of both managing problematic emotions and situations when they arise, by using a wide range of techniques derived from CBT, and understanding why it is that self-harm and other behaviours that may be considered impulsive are used by people with a history of trauma.

For young people who have self-harmed several times, consider offering developmental group psychotherapy with other young people. This should include at least six sessions but can be extended by mutual agreement (NICE 2004)

Depending on what is found at assessment, family therapy may also be indicated as a way of improving specific cognitive and social skills to promote the sharing of feelings, emotional control, and negotiation between family members.

The situation is more complex where there is an absence of defined mental health problems but where there are chronic problems relating to the environment, such as placement issues, schooling problems and family discord. In these circumstances the young person and the family may have expectations that mental health professionals can bring about change in these areas when this may not be the case. If school problems, particularly bullying, are prominent, liaison with the school is important. Further help may be provided by a school counsellor. In the case of learning difficulties, an assessment by an educational psychologist may be helpful in devising suitable educational options.

When the self-harm occurs alongside substance and alcohol misuse or violence, specific treatments for these conditions may be indicated. For older adolescents, referral to a self-help agency or walk-in counselling service may be appropriate – and more readily accepted (Hawton and James 2005).

Key points about self-harm

1. Self-harm is a behaviour that can occur in many different disorders and situations.

2. All self-harm needs assessment.

3. Self-harm in young people usually reflects acute distress and is usually not indicative of mental illness, in which case social, behavioural and psychotherapeutic approaches are advised.

4. Where there is an underlying mental illness, this should be appropriately treated as it will help reduce risk of further self-harm.

References

Centers for Disease Control (1990) 'Attempted Suicide among High School Students – United States.' *Journal of the American Medical Association 266*, 14, 1911–1912.

Hawton, K., Fagg, J. and Simkin, S. (1996) 'Deliberate self-poisoning and self-injury in children and adolescents under 16 years of age in Oxford, 1976–1993.' *British Journal of Psychiatry 169*, 202–208.

Hawton, K. and James, A. (2005) 'Suicide and deliberate self-harm in young people.' *British Medical Journal 330*, 891–894.

Hawton, K., Rodham, K., Evans, E. and Weatherall, R. (2002) 'Deliberate self-harm in adolescents: Self-report survey in schools in England.' *British Medical Journal 325*, 1207–1211.

Linehan, M. (1993) *Cognitive-Behavior Therapy for Borderline Personality Disorder.* New York: Guilford Press.

NICE Clinical Guideline 16 (2004) *Self-harm – The short-term physical and psychological management and secondary prevention of self-harm in primary and secondary care.* London: National Institute of Clinical Excellence. Available at www.nice.org.uk/page.aspx?o=cg016niceguideline, accessed on 14 December 2007.

Royal Australian and New Zealand College of Psychiatrists (2005) *Self-harm: Australian treatment guide for consumers and carers.* Available at http://dev.ranzcp.org/images/stories/ranzcp-attachments/pdfs/cpgs/AUS_CPGs/Self%20harm%20(Aus).pdf, accessed on 18 July 2008.

Websites

www.brightplace.org.uk/sh.html (Bright charity partnership)

www.focusas.com (Focus Adolescent Services)

www.selfharm.org.uk (Young People and Self-Harm)

www.nshn.co.uk (National Self-Harm Network)

www.suicidology.org (American Association of Suicidology)

www.afsp.org (American Foundation for Suicide Prevention)

CHAPTER 12

Mental Health Disorders

Depression

There has been increasing evidence over the last three decades that depression occurs in childhood and adolescence. Depression in children and young people should be seen as a spectrum of presentations which can range from mild to severe. Figures are very variable but a range of studies suggest that severe depression has a prevalence of 2–3 per cent in adolescence, whilst the prevalence is between 5 and 15 per cent for moderate depression. The prevalence of depression in childhood is lower than for adolescence with rates around 2.5 per cent, although twice that number may be significantly distressed (Birmaher, Ryan and Williamson 1996; Fombonne 1994; Kashani *et al.* 1987; Office for National Statistics 2000; 2005).

PRESENTATION

Young people may present with low mood as the primary complaint (this must be pervasive over time for depression to be diagnosed) or they may present with irritability instead, as well as a range of biological, affective and cognitive symptoms of depression including:

- changes in behaviour
- self-harm or thoughts about self-harm
- feelings of hopelessness
- negative self-image and low self-esteem
- losing interest and enjoyment in usual hobbies
- reduced motivation or enthusiasm

- reduced energy and readily fatigued
- poor concentration
- sleep problems (e.g. waking early, usually unfreshed)
- reduced appetite
- weight loss or failure to achieve expected weight gain
- inability to keep up at school
- frequent vague, non-specific physical symptoms, such as headache or tiredness
- an increase in moody, irritable, snappy, aggressive and hostile behaviour (often noted by parents)
- reduced emotional reactivity.

They may also present with features of disorders that are commonly comorbid with depression, such as anxiety, obsessions and compulsions. It is less common for young people to present with biological features. In severe depression the young person may additionally present with psychosis and have delusions of a nihilistic, self-derogatory or persecutory nature or hallucinations that support the young person's negative perception of tremendous feelings of worthlessness and hopelessness.

Whilst many young people report low mood, it is less clear how many have a mood disorder. Younger children may not have the vocabulary to articulate their feelings and they may choose to describe low mood when they are bored or understimulated or vice versa. Low mood is common in young people, but depression or a depressive illness is much less common. Signs of depression may be missed or incorrectly attributed to the perceived normal turmoil of adolescence. Outbursts, hostility and irritability may be interpreted as conduct disorder or disobedience. There needs to be a balance between not giving young people an inappropriate diagnosis and making sure a thorough assessment is undertaken to ensure treatable disorders are not missed.

RISK FACTORS
It is usually the interaction of several of the following risk factors that leads to depression.

- **Gender**

Prior to age 12 males report greater rates of depression, following which there is a reversal in the gender ratio. There is speculation that females may internalise their distress and report depression, whereas males externalise their distress, showing conduct disorder or substance use.

- **Self-image**

Poor self-esteem and negative body image are more common in females and may be antecedents of depression. There is currently no evidence to suggest that there is a neurochemical or hormonal basis for increased depression in females.

- **Family history**

There is a significantly increased risk of depression if one or both parents have a history of affective disorder. Marital and familial discord may increase the risk. Mother–child, father–child, parental and sibling relationships may also be factors in depression. Warm, communicative and caring parents instil confidence and high self-esteem in their children. A perception of parents as over-protective appears to be related to low levels of mastery and higher levels of depression. Parenting styles relate to adolescent self-esteem and low self-esteem can act as an antecedent for depression, as can parental rejection.

- **Attributional styles**

Social self-appraisal and self-esteem are important. Depressed young people tend to formulate faulty strategies to deal with social problems, and these are then aggravated by low self-esteem and low social confidence rendering them socially dysfunctional. Adolescents differentiate various domains of self-esteem and their evaluation of these appears to be linked to depression. Low self-perception about attractiveness and potential mates is linked to depression but not to scholastic, athletic or job domains. Stress may also be linked to depression.

- **Development and transitions**

Adolescents are susceptible to various stressors, such as biological changes, social changes (e.g. relocation), school transitions, parental separation, divorce or reconstitution of the family, and gender-role expectations.

- **Life events**

Accidents, bereavement, trauma, abuse and loss of romantic relationships.

- **Physical illness**

Especially chronic illness, such as diabetes and cystic fibrosis.

CONSEQUENCES OF DEPRESSION IN ADOLESCENCE

The most alarming consequence is suicide; however, depression alone is rarely the cause of suicide in adolescence. The other major consequence of depression in adolescence can be the interruption of the completion of developmental tasks in the educational, social and psychological spheres. Impairment in relationships with family and friends is a frequent feature of depression. The subsequent lack of social support may generate a negative feedback loop in which the consequences of the initial low mood may serve to maintain the depressive episode.

ASSESSMENT

If a young person is thought to be depressed they need to be assessed by a specialist service. Some primary care staff may be very good at recognising depression, but the majority are unlikely to have much experience of this. It is critical that a risk assessment is undertaken as part of the assessment.

MANAGEMENT

If a young person is expressing thoughts about self-harm and there is a high risk, inpatient management may be necessary until this feeling has subsided and the young person is more able to manage their feelings. If psychosis is present this needs treatment. Otherwise, in the first instance, counselling to address issues of self-esteem, social confidence, effective problem solving and managing relationships should be undertaken. If this is not effective after three sessions, then medication should be considered if criteria are met for a moderate or severe disorder. This should be done in conjunction with cognitive-behavioural therapy to address negative cognitions.

If the depression is related to past experiences, the issues around the experiences (such as abuse) will need to be addressed. Individual or group work to address issues of self-esteem, social confidence, effective problem solving and managing relationships may also need to be undertaken. The family will also need to be educated about the illness. Outcomes are usually good but likelihood of a recurrence is increased.

Case study: Tim

Tim is a 15-year-old boy with a three-month history of low mood (feeling sad), poor concentration, poor sleep, tiredness, lack of interest in playing football (he had been on his school team), with deterioration of his schoolwork. His parents felt he was also irritable and argumentative, which he had not been previously. They were also concerned with ideas of hopelessness although he had not considered self-harm. Tim eventually agrees to a referral to CAMHS.

What should the management plan include?

Psychosis

Psychosis is not a diagnosis in itself but a collection of signs that constitute a current mental state and indicate the presence of a physical cause or a 'functional' disorder such as schizophrenia or bipolar affective disorder (also known as manic-depression). Someone who is experiencing psychosis may have a range of signs or symptoms and these include:

- hallucinations – the experience of sensing something when there is not a real stimulus to that sensation; these may be auditory (e.g. hearing voices), visual, olfactory (smell), gustatory (taste), tactile or haptic (touch), or somatic (internal)

- delusions – firmly fixed, false beliefs that are not culturally contextual; these can be persecutory, nihilistic, religious, self-denigratory or grandiose in content

- thought disorder – including thought withdrawal, thought insertion, thought blocking ideas or delusions of passivity (that is the young person feels controlled by others or outside forces).

Another way that concern may be raised is if the young person shows a change in behaviour suggestive of paranoia, such as refusing to eat food prepared by someone in particular, or extreme responses to minor stimuli. These behaviours may be directly related to the perceptual abnormalities and thought disorder being experienced. The young person themselves may be very suspicious of interventions and often does not share everyone's concerns. In young people, common causes of psychosis are substance use, a medical cause (such as fever, trauma or epilepsy) or side-effects of prescribed medication. Psychosis may be associated with a mood disorder.

It may be difficult to differentiate between a true psychosis and a marked episode of derealisation or depersonalisation associated with acute anxiety or distress, particularly in children. A single short episode of psychosis does not necessarily mean that the young person has either an affective disorder or schizophrenia. Psychosis is more common in young people with a learning disability, including autism.

ASSESSMENT

Someone who is acutely psychotic needs urgent assessment and treatment. A risk assessment is important. Someone who has paranoid delusions may be at risk of harming others (believing they need to protect themselves) but they may also be a significant risk to themselves. This also applies to someone who is experiencing auditory hallucinations that may command them to harm themselves. As the person is unable to differentiate these perceptions from their normal ones, they may obey the hallucinations.

Assessment is required to establish whether the young person is psychotic, and this needs to be undertaken by specialist CAMHS. Assessment will also help identify the potential causes of the psychosis, including medical causes. The young person may be unable to give a competent history because of their mental state, so corroborative histories from other informants such as family members or teachers are important. It can be difficult to identify substance use, but for psychosis in adolescence this is a strong possibility. Urine and blood tests to detect substances may be appropriate. However, consent is required for this. A full assessment may thus take place over a period of days or weeks.

MANAGEMENT

Early intervention is essential and may comprise medication, specialist nursing, psychoeducation, provision of specialist milieu in the form of day hospital or inpatient care, and rehabilitation. As well as addressing associated risk, early intervention may improve prognosis (Lehman 2007). A person who is psychotic is likely to need admission, particularly where there is marked distress or risk and if antipsychotic medication is going to be administered. Unfortunately, the facilities to admit acutely psychotic young people to specialist adolescent units may be very limited. Adult wards, which should be avoided where possible, may sometimes be the only viable option, in which case it is crucial that young people receive appropriate support from child and adolescent mental health specialists.

Antipsychotic medication in young people can have significant side-effects that can last beyond the course of treatment, and the medication may need to be given under supervision. However, specialist community-based early psychosis intervention teams can deliver safe and effective treatment without the need for admission (McGorry and Jackson 1999). The early management needs to include the acute psychosis and allow investigation to establish a diagnosis so the underlying problem can be appropriately addressed.

Nursing care in the community or hospital plays an important part in supporting young people with psychoses: key features include engaging with the young person, reality orientation (in time, place and person) and provision of a calm, comfortable, secure and predictable environment that is non-excitatory.

Psychosis can be frightening for the young person and their family, so sensitive support is essential, which should include the provision of information about psychosis and its treatment. Irrespective of the cause of the psychosis, assessment should be made early on during treatment of the young person's needs following recovery. This will lead to the development of an agreed rehabilitation programme, which may include ongoing family and community support or alternative accommodation, clinical reviews, support in activities of daily living, and an individualised education programme or, in older teenagers, retraining and sheltered work experience. Rehabilitation depends on close cross-agency working between the mental health team and front-line professionals.

Bipolar affective disorder (manic-depressive disorder)

Bipolar affective disorder is rare in early adolescence or prepubertally (exact prevalence figures are generally not available) but can be very difficult to manage when it does occur. It is also commonly known as manic-depressive illness indicating each end of the bipolar spectrum.

PRESENTATION

A young person who has bipolar affective disorder is usually likely to first present with a depressive episode. The manic episode may appear during treatment of the depressive episode or after the depressive episode has resolved. A manic episode is characterised by:

- elated mood, although the mood is often very labile (that is changeable)
- being generally irritable with episodes of expansive and elated behaviour
- apparent boundless energy
- taking on a number of tasks, most of which will be left uncompleted
- poor concentration and attention
- little continuity of thought
- expression of a number of disconnected or tenuously connected ideas
- rapid speech and frustration at other people's inability to keep up
- expression of grandiose ideas and schemes
- making unrealistic and over-ambitious plans
- poor sleep
- disinhibition and engagement in socially and sexually inappropriate behaviour
- risk of engaging in unprotected and unwanted sexual activity
- risk of abuse because of increased vulnerability
- reduced likelihood to make competent decisions.

It may also be clinically difficult to differentiate bipolar affective disorder from schizophrenia at the time of the first episode because of the nature of the presentation.

RISK FACTORS

Family history of the disorder is the major risk factor, and whilst stress may trigger episodes it does not cause bipolar affective disorder.

ASSESSMENT

Urgent assessment may be required depending on the presentation. It is important to undertake a risk assessment, including issues of self-harm ideation and child protection, which may be a priority as some of the behaviours associated with bipolar affective disorder (e.g. disinhibition, hypersexuality) may put the young person at considerable risk.

MANAGEMENT

The acute phase of mania needs to be treated, and depending on social supports this may be managed at home. If the mania is moderate or severe, inpatient care is likely to be the most appropriate option. Young people can be very difficult to manage when they are acutely manic and often do not receive therapeutic doses of appropriate medication. Atypical antipsychotic medication is increasingly used to manage acute psychosis, although older medications may still be widely used. Mood stabilisers (such as lithium, sodium valproate) may be used in the acute phase together with antipsychotic medication and then continued as maintenance medication after a repeat episode. Rehabilitation should be considered as described under psychosis above.

Schizophrenia

Schizophrenia may be seen as a collection of several disorders rather than one single disease or illness. However, all the disorders have a degree of psychosis but some will have a greater degree of the negative signs and symptoms of the disorder as described below. It is important to understand that schizophrenia is not a 'split personality' as is sometimes thought. Schizophrenia is uncommon in early adolescence, but prevalence increases by late adolescence, especially in males (Torrey 1987). It may be that some of the 'odd young people' seen in early or mid adolescence are in a pre-illness or prodromal phase. In adults the prevalence of schizophrenia is 1 per cent internationally. It is significantly less than this in children and adolescents.

PRESENTATION

Young people may present:

- acutely in a psychotic state

- less acutely with delusions, thought disorder or hallucinations or more gradually with subtle changes in personality
- with a significant reduction in social contacts
- with deterioration in general and academic functioning
- with a reduction in personal care and hygiene.

Some young people present with what are called 'negative signs' such as:

- decreased functioning in multiple areas (e.g. socially, academically)
- blunted or flat affect, or inappropriate responses of emotion
- reduced energy or spontaneity (avolition)
- lack of enjoyment (anhedonia).

Young people may not understand or agree with their parents that there is anything wrong and may be very suspicious and dismissive of efforts made to engage them. They may appear to present with other conditions when the presentation is gradual.

RISK FACTORS

Family history is a recognised risk factor in schizophrenia and individuals with schizophrenia are also more likely to have:

- a family history with increased risk if there is a diagnosis in a first-degree relative (i.e. parent, sibling) or in multiple relatives
- biochemical factors – in that individuals with schizophrenia appear to have a neurochemical imbalance of some neurotransmitters
- altered brain structure and function – for example, people with schizophrenia appear to have difficulty coordinating activity between different areas of the brain (shown by using positron emission tomography (PET) scans) and the ventricles of people with schizophrenia are often enlarged (shown by using magnetic resonance imaging (MRI) scans) (Johnstone *et al.* 1978).

Some factors, whilst not necessarily causing schizophrenia, can perpetuate an episode or trigger relapse:

- stress

- substance use – although there is increasing evidence of a potentially causal link between cannabis use and schizophrenia

- family communication – family-based interventions can reduce relapse in families that express high levels of emotion (Kavanagh 1992; Vaughn and Leff 1976).

ASSESSMENT

Any young person presenting with acute psychosis needs urgent assessment as discussed above. However, the presentation in young people is often more gradual and less clear. There may be non-specific concerns about the young person being odd (e.g. inappropriate social responses), a loner or beginning to withdraw socially. If the presentation is unclear, the assessment may need to be completed over a few months and any changes carefully monitored. Schizophrenia may also coexist with a mood disorder.

MANAGEMENT

In addition to the general management of psychosis described above, there are several areas that need to be addressed in a young person with schizophrenia:

- **Longer-term management of psychosis and the maintenance of medication**

This also needs to include strategies to reduce the distress that is often associated with hallucinations, for example diversionary tactics, relaxation techniques and recreational activities.

- **Individual cognitive-behavioural therapy**

This is needed to help develop skills and appropriate coping strategies.

- **Education of the young person and their family about the disorder**

It may also be helpful to consider the impact of the illness on the family and the range of emotions the family members may experience once a diagnosis has been made. Feelings may include anger, guilt, shame, sadness, a sense of loss, isolation and ambivalence. The family may find itself under considerable stress and need support in their own right. Self-help and family support groups through national or local organisations may be the most useful way of addressing this. The family may also need to be educated about possible relapses and the need for early interventions.

- **Social support and rehabilitation**
This may be through group or individual work. It also needs to address the issues of rehabilitating the young person into society especially if they have had a lengthy period of illness. They may lack confidence as well as face considerable prejudice. Recreational opportunities are also important. Peer support may be especially important for young people.

Unfortunately, the side-effects of some of the medications used to manage psychotic illnesses are more marked in young people and are significantly distressing, making compliance difficult. These issues need to be sensitively and carefully addressed with the young person.

Eating disorders in older children and adolescents
Young people are often dissatisfied with their appearance and their attempt to change it can result in an eating disorder. Worries about weight, shape, food and dieting are especially common amongst teenage girls. The majority of problems occur in young people between the ages of 14 and 19 years. Eating disorders, such as anorexia nervosa and bulimia nervosa, occur more frequently in girls but have more recently started to increase in

---

Case study: Simon
Simon is a 16-year-old boy coming up to doing his GCSEs. Until six months ago he had been making plans enthusiastically for a career in business and had decided which A-levels he wanted to take. However, over the last six months there has been a gradual deterioration in his socialisation. His mother notes that he appears to have become particularly selfish, not being interested in what other members of the family want or need. He will often insist on watching a television programme and get very angry if he is not allowed to watch what he wants. The family have found that they have tended to give in to this because it avoids a confrontation. However, they have noted that even when he is

---

watching television he will sometimes look quite blank, while at other times he can appear quite agitated. He will often not participate in family conversations although will misinterpret what is said.

Simon's parents come and meet with you to express their concerns. How would you manage this?

After some persuasion, Simon agrees to meet with you. What are the key areas that you would need to ask Simon about?

Simon is subsequently seen at a CAMHS. After a time a diagnosis of schizophrenia is made on the basis of the history and mental state examinations. The assessment is completed by a brief admission to hospital. Simon is started on risperidone and after a couple of weeks' hospitalisation is discharged from hospital.

What roles do the school and the GP have in supporting Simon's rehabilitation?

What cultural issues might there be?

---

boys. These disorders are ten times more common in girls than boys with the prevalence rate for girls between 15 and 19 years being around 1 per cent (Crisp, Palmer and Kalucy 1976); however, rates are variable across different populations. Studies across the globe show rates of 0.69 per cent in Spain (Morande, Celada and Casas 1999), 0.7 per cent in Switzerland (Steinhausen, Winkler and Meier 1997), 0.84 per cent in Sweden (Rastam, Gillberg and Garton 1989). In non-Western populations it may be that there are different variants of the disorder (Srinivasan, Suresh and Jayaram 1998) although one Iranian study found rates that were comparable to Western populations (Nobakht and Dezhkam 2000). Rates are often higher in private educational facilities (Rastam *et al.* 1989), ballet dancers and models.

Anorexia nervosa

A young person with anorexia nervosa nearly always starts by restricting dietary intake ('dieting'). Around one-third have been overweight before starting to diet. Although 'anorexia' literally means 'loss of appetite', the appetite is usually normal and the usual hunger cues misinterpreted.

PRESENTATION

The young person may present with the following:

- marked distortion of body image such that the person believes themselves to be overweight when they are not

- marked weight loss – body weight is consistently 15 per cent less (or lower) than that expected for height and age, or body mass index is 17.5 or less; this can be due to either weight loss, or failure to gain weight during growth

- a preoccupation with thinness or dieting

- an intense fear of being fat or of calories

- preoccupation with food, for example often prepares food for others

- continuing to diet when thin

- compulsive exercising

- lying about food

- self-induced vomiting or use of laxatives

- denial of a problem

- physical development interrupted or hindered

- irregularities or cessation of menstrual cycle (three missed cycles if menstruation was established)

- hair loss

- cold extremities

- growth of a fine, downy hair all over the body

- dental decay

- depression

- anxiety.

RISK FACTORS

Young people may feel under considerable social pressure to conform to current fashion trends, media images of attractiveness and peer pressures. However, the risk of developing anorexia is more likely in the presence of the following factors:

- feeling of not being in control in one or many aspects of their lives; dieting can be a tangible way of showing self-control

- fear of growing up or developing (puberty)

- poor communication or self expression in the family or over-protectiveness or criticism within the family

- personality characteristics of over-compliance, perfectionism, and dependence

- family history of anorexia nervosa (though some research findings are conflicting)

- stressful life events (including loss, threats to self-integrity, and physical illness).

ASSESSMENT

It is usually parents or friends who become concerned, and assessment can be difficult as the young person is often resistant to hearing that there are valid concerns for their safety. It is important to undertake a full mental health and physical health history. The impact of starvation has physical implications, which if not recognised or managed may have serious consequences. Vital signs (temperature, blood pressure and pulse) should be recorded at first interview. Complications of the disorder include muscle weakness, heart murmurs, tooth decay, bowel damage, kidney damage, seizures, loss of bone density, gastric ulcers, coma and death. Studies on the mortality rate of young people with anorexia suggest that it is high: between 5 per cent (Neumaker 1997; Sullivan 1995) and 10 per cent. If there is rapid weight loss, then urgent medical assessment and treatment is necessary.

MANAGEMENT

It is easier to help young people if the problem is noticed and dealt with early. The more entrenched the problem the more difficult it is to manage. Problems are usually recognised by the family, so they can be important in the assessment and treatment of the problem. The first step to treating an eating disorder is recognising it.

Once the problem is suspected or recognised, referral to CAMHS is necessary. Depending on the severity of the condition, there may be a need

Case study: Nasreen

Nasreen is a 15-year-old girl who has a four-month history of weight loss and changing body image. She has been exercising excessively as she feels that she remains too fat despite the recent weight loss. As her schoolteacher, you have become increasingly concerned as she is looking thinner. She is often cold and unable to concentrate. You are worried that Nasreen may have anorexia nervosa and encourage her to seek help. Nasreen insists that there is nothing wrong.

How would you manage the situation?

Can the school use the Mental Health Act to get Nasreen to see a mental health professional?

Nasreen is taken to the GP by her mother and referred to CAMHS, where a diagnosis of anorexia nervosa is confirmed.

What might be the specific cultural issues that need to be considered in this case?

for the intervention to take place in an inpatient setting. Eating disorders such as anorexia can often make it difficult for the young person to take part in regular family life; therefore, it is important to support the family through the intervention as well.

If there are several different professionals involved in the care it is imperative that there be a single cohesive management plan that addresses all components of the young person's health. The very nature of the problem means that the young person has distorted cognitions, so they can present as hostile and uncooperative. It may be useful to see this as an expression of their difficulty in managing the situation. It is crucial to involve the family collaboratively in the management to minimise the possibility of miscommunication and ensure the parents continue to take responsibility as appropriate.

The general principles of management and treatment include:

- encouraging regular, balanced meals in consultation with a dietician

- directing therapies at the young person's self-image, including body image and self-esteem, and helping to cope with peer influence

- achieving a balanced exercise regime
- ensuring sufficient sleep and rest
- encouraging the young person not to be influenced by other people skipping meals or commenting on weight
- achieving gradual weight gain
- engaging in concurrent individual and/or family therapy, depending on underlying issues; family therapy is the treatment of choice for young people with anorexia nervosa under 15 years of age.

Bulimia nervosa

Bulimia often consists of binge eating or consumption of excessive amounts of high-calorie food over a short space of time. Purging often follows this, which is associated with immense feelings of guilt for having consumed 'restricted' foods. This disorder is seen in older adolescents and adults, and is uncommon in younger children.

PRESENTATION

Bulimia is characterised by:

- a fear of fatness
- binge eating: there is a constant obsession with eating and the overwhelming desire for food leads to episodes of eating large amounts of food in short time periods
- maintenance of normal weight
- purging by vomiting and/or excessive use of laxatives
- alternating episodes of calorie restriction, using appetite suppressants, or diuretics
- feeling out of control
- depression or mood swings.

Complications of bulimia can include swollen glands in the face and neck from vomiting, weakness and exhaustion, damage to bowels from taking laxatives, and stomach acid may dissolve the enamel on teeth.

In many cases, the bulimia follows an episode of anorexia nervosa, although the period of time between the two disorders may vary considerably.

MANAGEMENT

As with anorexia nervosa the following are useful:

- encouraging regular, balanced meals in consultation with a dietician

- directing therapies at the young person's self-image, including body image and self-esteem, and helping to cope with peer influence

- achieving a balanced exercise regime

- psychoeducation about healthy eating.

Cognitive-behavioural techniques (including diary keeping) are particularly useful. The outcome for bulimia is generally good in the absence of other problems.

Substance use and problem substance use (PSU)

Substance misuse can be harmful to young people in a number of ways. It can threaten their health and welfare, and prevent them from reaching their full potential across a number of domains. Substance misuse in young people is widespread, but can be preventable (McKay, Hatton and McDougall 2006). For most people who use psychoactive ('mind-altering') drugs, their first experience was in adolescence. There is generally positive promotion of alcohol and tobacco with a strong cultural ambivalence with respect to other drugs. It is difficult to be precise about the prevalence of substance use as much of the information is usually self-reported by young people. However, in the UK, it has been estimated that one in ten young people between the ages of 11 and 15 years uses drugs at some point (HAS 2001). In recent years there has been an escalation of use in many countries including the UK and Australia (Miller and Plant 1996; National Statistics 2000; Success Works 1998; Sutherland and Willner 1998). These studies also show that over the years the gender divide has decreased, as has the age at first use. Miller and Plant (1996) found cigarette smoking to be more common among girls than boys. A follow-up study found that whilst alcohol and cigarette use remained stable, illicit drug use had fallen suggesting that this may have reached a temporary saturation point (Miller and Plant 2001). Whilst use during adolescence may not be problem use, it may lead to tangible problems in the future. Young people who use substances are more likely to:

- be involved in road traffic and other accidents
- find their psychological and emotional development impaired
- have coexisting mental health problems
- self-harm and attempt or complete suicide
- be involved in crime, including murder (as victims and perpetrators)
- contract sexually transmitted diseases (through unprotected sex as they may be disinhibited and less cognitively aware, or may also be sexually active to fund drug taking)
- be homeless
- be at increased risk of contracting HIV through shared needle use.

A wider range of drugs is now available for use. There is also increased polydrug use (i.e. the use of more than one drug).

RISK FACTORS
Risk factors for problem substance use fall into three categories: environmental, individual and family.

Environmental factors

- access and drug availability
- peer influence and social acceptance
- social status (any marginalised group may be at increased risk)
- poor community networks.

Individual factors

- psychiatric comorbidity (depression, anxiety, conduct disorder, psychosis and ADHD)
- genetic/biological predisposition
- psychological factors such as personality characteristics, ability to cope.

Family factors

- chaotic families
- families with mental health problems
- families that have a substance use history
- abuse
- how the family handles adolescence and the issues that it brings
- families with relationship problems.

TYPES OF DRUGS USED

The same drug will often have a wide variety of names, and just as professionals become streetwise with the current names, so they keep changing. Professionals need to keep themselves updated if they work in this area. Within local groups and contexts there may also be different names used. Many substances have more than one effect and may be used for any of the effects. Commonly used substances are shown in Figure 12.1. Although not used for psychoactive purposes, anabolic steroids can also impact on mental health.

MANAGEMENT

Brief intervention may be appropriate for young people with less serious problem substance use. However, it can be a mistake to assume that young people cannot have serious PSU as the major issue. Interventions aimed at risk reduction have been found to be the most effective in improving morbidity. This can include abstinence, though this does not need to be a goal, except for high-risk substance use such as solvent and petrol sniffing. Whilst young people should not be given the impression that professionals

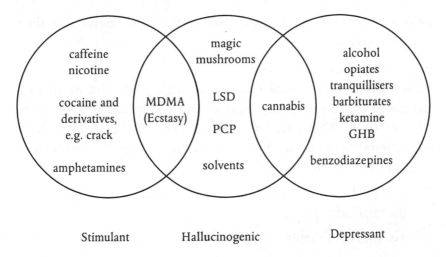

Figure 12.1 The psychoactive effects of drugs commonly used

condone their substance use, they also should not feel criticised or judged as this is unlikely to engage them. If they remain engaged, they are more likely to return and seek help at a later stage.

Management includes:

- **Education**

Providing accurate information on substances and how to use them safely may help to minimise harm. This can be very controversial, as some feel that giving young people information and not judging their substance use condones such behaviour. Young people are likely to use drugs if that is what they have decided, and minimising further risks such as pregnancy and sexually transmitted diseases (through unprotected sex if uninhibited and judgement impaired), may be the best, if not the only, option. Most individuals are ambivalent about change, and young substance users are no exception.

- **Motivational Interviewing**

Motivational Interviewing techniques (a brief psychotherapeutic intervention), which use focused and goal directed approaches to bring about change in the person, have proven successful in working with young people who misuse drugs and alcohol. Over a period of time, it can help to instigate a desire to change any negative behaviours, and help the young person to explore any feelings of ambivalence their may have (NICE 2007).

• **Family-based interventions**

Family-based interventions can also be highly effective in offering structured support to young people who are involved in substance misuse (NICE 2007). Engagement of a family member in the delivery of any intervention is the single most positive prognostic factor. Such interventions would include:

1. at least three motivational interview sessions with parents/carers

2. assessment of family interaction

3. parenting skills training

4. encouraging parents to monitor their child's behaviour and academic performance

5. offering feedback to the family on progress

6. more intensive support offered to families who are found to need it.

• **Monitoring**

If, through monitoring, the young person is able to see their substance use increasing, and see problems arising from it, they may be more motivated to begin to change their life.

• **Medically assisted withdrawal**

Medically assisted withdrawal is usually best done in a safe and supportive environment, although increasingly home-based withdrawals may be considered. During withdrawal, as well as medication, relaxation techniques, massages, exercise and emotional support may be of help.

• **Rehabilitation**

May include maintenance drug programmes (again these can be very controversial for young people), recreational activities, as well as other components of rehabilitation listed under psychosis above. This can prove difficult in economically and socially disadvantaged areas.

References

Birmaher, B., Ryan, N.D. and Williamson, D.E. (1996) 'Childhood and adolescent depression: A review of the past ten years. Part 1.' *Journal of the American Academy of Child and Adolescent Psychiatry 35*, 11, 1427–1439.

Crisp, A.H., Palmer, R.L. and Kalucy, R.S. (1976) 'How common is anorexia? A prevalence study.' *British Journal of Psychiatry 128*, 549–554.

Fombonne, E. (1994) 'Increased rates of depression: Update of epidemiological findings and analytical problems.' *Acta Psychiatrica Scandinavica 90*, 3, 145–156.

Health Advisory Service (2001) *The Substance of Young Needs: A Review.* London: Health Advisory Service.

Johnstone, E.C., Crow, T.J., Frith, C.D., Stevens, M., Kreel, L. and Husband, J. (1978) 'The dementia of dementia praecox.' *Acta Psychiatrica Scandinavia 57*, 305–324.

Kashani, J.H., Beck, N.C., Hoeper, E.W., Fallahi, C. *et al.* (1987) 'Psychiatric disorders in a community sample of adolescents.' *American Journal of Psychiatry 144*, 584–589.

Kavanagh, D.J. (1992) 'Recent developments in expressed emotion and schizophrenia.' In J. Jenkins, K. Oatley and N. Stein (eds) (1998) *Human Emotions – A Reader.* London: Blackwell Publications.

Lehman, A.F. (2007) 'Early intervention for psychosis and schizophrenia.' *Journal of Nervous and Mental Disease 195*, 12, 965–967.

McGorry, P.D. and Jackson, H.J. (1999) *The Recognition and Management of Early Psychosis: A Preventative Approach.* Cambridge: Cambridge University Press.

McKay, D., Hatton, T. and McDougall, T. (2006) 'Substance misuse, young people and nursing.' In T. McDougall (ed.) *Child and Adolescent Mental Health Nursing.* London: Blackwell Publications.

Miller, P. and Plant, M.A. (1996) 'Drinking, smoking, and illicit drug use among 15- and 16-year-olds in the United Kingdom.' *British Medical Journal 313*, 394–397.

Miller, P. and Plant, M.A. (2001) 'Drinking and smoking among 15- and 16-year-olds in the United Kingdom: A re-examination.' *Journal of Substance Use 5*, 4, 285–289.

Morande, G., Celada, J. and Casas, J.J. (1999) 'Prevalence of eating disorders in a Spanish school-age population.' *Journal of Adolescent Health 24*, 3, 212–219.

National Statistics (2000) *Statistical Bulletin: Statistics on Young People and Drug Misuse: England 1998.* London: Department of Health.

Neumaker, K.J. (1997) 'Mortality and sudden death in anorexia nervosa.' *International Journal of Eating Disorders 21*, 3, 205–212.

NICE (2007) *Interventions to Reduce Substance Misuse among Vulnerable Young People.* London: NICE.

Nobakht, M. and Dezhkam, M. (2000) 'An epidemiological study of eating disorders in Iran.' *International Journal of Eating Disorders 28*, 3, 265–271.

Office for National Statistics (2000) *Mental Health of Children and Adolescents in Great Britain.* London: The Stationery Office.

Office for National Statistics (2005) *Mental Health of Children and Young People in Great Britain, 2004.* Basingstoke: Palgrave McMillan.

Rastam, M., Gillberg, C. and Garton, M. (1989) 'Anorexia nervosa in a Swedish urban region: A population-based study.' *British Journal of Psychiatry 155*, 642–646.

Srinivasan, T.N., Suresh, T.R. and Jayaram, V. (1998) 'Emergence of eating disorders in India: Study of eating distress syndrome and development of a screening questionnaire.' *International Journal of Social Psychiatry 44*, 3, 189–198.

Steinhausen, H.C., Winkler, C. and Meier, M. (1997) 'Eating disorders in adolescence in a Swiss epidemiological study.' *International Journal of Eating Disorders 22*, 2, 147–151.

Success Works Pty Ltd (1998) *Young People and Drugs: Needs Analysis.* Melbourne Department of Human Services, State Government of Victoria.

Sullivan, P.F. (1995) 'Mortality in anorexia nervosa.' *American Journal of Psychiatry 152*, 7, 1073–1074.

Sutherland, I. and Willner, P. (1998) 'Patterns of alcohol, cigarette and illicit drug use in English adolescents.' *Addiction 93*, 1199–1208.

Torrey, E.F. (1987) 'Prevalence studies in schizophrenia.' *British Journal of Psychiatry 150*, 598–608.

Vaughn, C.E. and Leff, J.P. (1976) 'Influence of family and social factors on the course of psychiatric illness.' *British Journal of Psychiatry 129*, 125.

Further reading

Bryant Waugh, R. and Lask, B. (1999) *Eating Disorder: A Parents' Guide*. London: Penguin.

Emmett, D. and Nice, G. (2005) *Understanding Drug Issues: A Photocopiable Resource Workbook* (2nd edition). London: Jessica Kingsley Publishers.

Garner, D.M. and Garfinkel, P.E. (eds) (1997) *Handbook and Treatment of Eating Disorders*. London: Guilford Press.

Graham, P. and Hughes, C. (1995) *So Sad, So Young, So Listen*. London: Royal College of Psychiatrists and Gaskell.

McGorry, P.D., Yung, A.R., Bechdolf, A. and Amminger, P. (2008) 'Back to the future: Predicting and reshaping the course of psychotic disorder.' *Archives of General Psychiatry 65*, 25–27.

NICE (2002) *Self-harm: The Short Term Physical and Psychological Management and Secondary Preventions of Self-harm in Primary and Secondary Care*. London: NICE.

NICE (2004) *Eating Disorders: Core Interventions in the Treatment of Anorexia Nervosa, Bulimia Nervosa and Other Related Eating Disorders*. London: NICE.

NICE (2005) *Depression in Children and Young People: Identification and Management in Primary Care, Community and Secondary Care*. London: NICE.

NTA (2007) *Assessing Young People for Substance Misuse*. London: NTA. Available at www.nta.nhs.uk/publications/documents/nta_assessing_young__people__for__substance __misuse_yp1.pdf, accessed on 18 July 2008.

Pagliaro, A.M. and Pagliaro, L.A. (1996) *Substance Use Among Children and Adolescents: Its Nature, Extent and Effects from Conception to Adulthood*. Chichester: Wiley.

Palmer, B. (2000) *Helping People with Eating Disorders*. London: Wiley.

Royal College of Psychiatrists (1982) 'The management of parasuicide in young people under sixteen: Report from the Child and Adolescent Section.' *Bulletin of the Royal College of Psychiatrists* October, 182–185.

Royal College of Psychiatrists (1998) *Managing deliberate self-harm in young people*. (Council Report CR 64). London: Royal College of Psychiatrists.

Torrey, E.F. (1996) *Surviving Schizophrenia: A Manual for Families, Consumers and Providers* (3rd edition). New York: HarperCollins.

Websites

www.adf.org.au (Australian Drug Foundation)
www.eatingdisorderscentre.co.uk (Eating Disorders Centre)
www.mind.org.uk (Mind)
www.nimh.nih.gov (National Institute of Mental Health, US)
www.nta.nhs.uk (National Treatment Agency for Substance Misuse)
www.rcpsych.ac.uk (Royal College of Psychiatrists)

See also Royal College of Psychiatrists fact sheets, available through the Royal College on a range of mental health problems.

PART 5

Treatment and Management Strategies

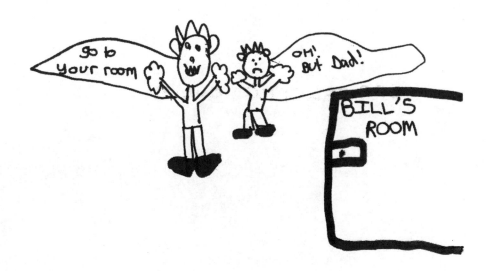

CHAPTER 13

Basic Interventions with Applicability in Primary Care Settings

Planning interventions

Before an appropriate intervention can be planned, there should be a full and thorough assessment as described earlier. Intervention can then be discussed and agreed with the young person and the family. The first need is to decide which type of therapy is appropriate, whether this should be individual, group or family based, and whether medication is required. This needs to be written in a management plan with clear ideas of when the situation is to be reviewed. No treatment should be unplanned or open-ended. If the treatment does not lead to resolution, reconsider the diagnosis or formulation of the problem. It is important not to continue treatment that does not improve matters without reviewing the situation. Professionals should ensure they use the appropriate strategy for the identified problem rather than using a single strategy, technique or approach for all problems. The strategies discussed in this chapter have particular applicability in primary care; but, additionally, the usefulness of education, support and listening provided by adults should not be underestimated.

Management of complex problems

The management of mental health problems can be complicated by other health and social needs. These include serious or chronic medical disorders, such as epilepsy, and social needs, such as provision of alternative care or educational needs. Where issues of management interact, it is important for the various agencies to work closely together. It is important that those working with complex needs start to try to understand and gain knowledge surrounding young people's mental health problems, in order to identify them early. Sometimes significant mental health problems are missed, or parents are not prepared for what they may have to cope with. These difficulties can often lead to breakdown in placement.

As the nature of these young people's difficulties is often complex, the provision for their mental health problems must take place collaboratively. It is vital for all agencies involved to work together. Recently some CAMHS have developed services specifically for young people at high risk of complex needs. However, for these to be effective there still must be a great deal of planning and partnership.

Interventions can occur at a number of levels:

- through local networks of services meeting together to plan responsive services

- through social workers and parents accessing consultation offered by local CAMHS

- in multi-agency training initiatives

- through the development of support groups, with local CAMHS professionals involved, where parents and professionals can work together to approach problems consistently and strategically

- through a range of therapeutic interventions in a multi-agency setting, to meet specific needs and problems (e.g. post-abuse services, substance misuse services, youth offending teams and the voluntary sector).

Behaviour therapy
What behaviour therapy is and is not

Behaviour therapy is one application of behavioural theories and works on the principle that the frequency of a given behaviour can be increased or decreased by modifying stimuli that influence it. These stimuli can be therapeutically manipulated, either by the person showing the behaviour or by someone else, who in the case of young people may be a parent or teacher. Behaviour therapy can be used in a variety of conditions across the life span: anxiety disorders (such as phobia, social anxiety and separation anxiety), obsessive-compulsive disorder, enuresis (wetting) and encopresis (soiling), behaviour and conduct disorders, and behavioural aspects of psychotic disorders.

Parents or young people may seek an answer to the question *why* a behaviour occurs. Even if there were an answer to this question, the identified behaviour would be unlikely to change. Improved insight does not necessarily result in a change in behaviour, and vice versa. Behaviour therapy is not an insight-directed therapy nor a punitive approach to social control. Punishment (by an individual, organisation or society) is the least effective way to bring about change, and usually has more to do with making those in control feel better or being least inconvenienced. Criticisms of behaviour therapy are usually based on confusion between these issues, or on the notion that an individual's thoughts and feelings are ignored, which would not be good practice. Behaviour therapy should always benefit the individual and not be used to allow others to exercise control. These ethical considerations are particularly important in the most vulnerable, such as young people with learning disability.

The application of behavioural theories

Classical conditioning, operant conditioning, social learning theory and cognitive learning are described in Chapter 4. These are directly relevant to treatment. In practice, two or more models come into play in the expression of behaviour and in treatment. For instance, a child who receives little parental attention may frequently show antisocial history, the consequence of which is to be told off – which, however unpleasant, is still the attention desired. This illustrates both social learning theory and operant conditioning. The treatment of a phobia by systematic desensitisation to the feared object involves both conditioning to a new stimulus (classical conditioning) and the reward of decreased anxiety while in the continued presence of the feared object (positive reinforcement of operant conditioning).

Behaviour therapy in practice

Behaviour therapy is often part of an overall management of a disorder or identified problem. It should only be considered after a comprehensive assessment has been made. It is unlikely to be the only intervention. Behaviour therapy can be successfully implemented in primary care as well as in specialist services, providing the professional has had relevant training and receives appropriate supervision.

Behaviour therapy may be undertaken individually (with parents or young people), or with families, or in therapeutic groups (for parents or young people). Whatever the mode of delivery, the principles remain the same. Some parent training groups provide general education about the use of behavioural approaches using the same principles. There are four components to its implementation, as outlined here:

- engagement
- defining goals
- assessment of the behaviour
- implementation and follow-through.

ENGAGEMENT

This entails that everyone understands what the purpose of the intervention is and is motivated to carry it out. As a strong commitment of time and energy over several weeks or months is required, the family need to be active participants in planning the management. The family should be informed of the nature and purpose of behaviour therapy and agree to it. They may accept that it is appropriate but have other more pressing issues to address first, or may need to spend time preparing themselves, in which instances the programme should be postponed.

DEFINING GOALS

Once engaged, the parents or young person, or both, should identify which behaviour(s) they wish to change. This usually concerns reducing or stopping undesirable behaviour. Goals should be specific, definable and achievable. A parent's request that their child should 'be good and not behave badly' or a young person's request 'not to worry about things' does not meet these criteria for goals. Such requests need to be explored further and specific behaviours identified (e.g. 'to stop hitting his brother' or 'to mix with friends without feeling anxious'). It is often prudent to start with the most dangerous examples of behaviour first, or with those that may be most readily addressed. The goal may have to be broken down into several achievable steps.

Reducing the frequency of an undesirable behaviour is more readily achieved and maintained if a desired behaviour with which it is incompatible is simultaneously encouraged. For example a child who is encouraged to play happily with his brother cannot be hitting him at the same time; the more he remains engaged in play, the less he will hit. It is important to build in rewards for the desired behaviour as well as trying to extinguish the undesired behaviour. Sometimes parents first want to see their child showing an improved 'attitude' or 'respect', which is variably defined. However, these are less tangible, and changes at this level follow changes in behaviour rather than the other way round.

ASSESSMENT OF THE BEHAVIOUR

The assessment of the identified behaviour(s) should entail a systematic examination of the influences on that behaviour. This includes a careful history and a *functional analysis*, which is a detailed breakdown of antecedents, behaviour and consequences (ABC). These can be recorded on an 'ABC chart' over a period of time that would give sufficient examples to work with clinically. The chart may be completed by the young person themselves, if appropriate, or an informant, who may be a parent, carer or teacher. It may be necessary for the professional to make direct observations of the child and their environment in the same way, or use videotaped examples. The chart is usually in the form shown in Figure 13.1 below, with observation of the factors in italics described in each column.

Date / time	A (antecedents)	B (behaviour)	C (consequences)
	Where? *With whom?* *What was the child doing?* *What were others doing?*	*Nature / type of behaviour – described in detail.* *Duration?* *Severity?*	*What did the child do afterwards?* *What did others do afterwards?* *Were there any changes in attention given to, and in expectations of, the child?*

Figure 13.1 An 'ABC chart' used in the functional analysis of behaviour

Adolescents with phobic disorder can use the same chart to identify the specific influences on their avoidant behaviour. Whatever the identified problem, it is sometimes helpful to have more than one person completing charts of the same events if possible. One person may observe an aspect of the situation that others do not.

IMPLEMENTATION AND FOLLOW-THROUGH

The stimuli to the undesired behaviour identified by the functional analysis can be avoided and the most appropriate techniques to encourage desired behaviour identified. (see Table 13.1 for a list of common techniques.) It is helpful to discuss the use and value of different techniques and what the parent or young person has already tried, and how. The analysis may demonstrate an inconsistent approach by parents, which is common. If the child has been unable to predict the consequences of particular behaviours, the hoped-for reduction in undesirable behaviour cannot be achieved. Parents may be inconsistent with each other or one parent may be inconsistent over time. The need for consistency should be emphasised in the programme devised. Parents may have an over-reliance on techniques that are least potent or have only short-term effects (such as shouting, nagging, slapping), while neglecting more reliable techniques because of previous inconsistency in their implementation. This should be carefully evaluated and discussed with the parent.

Time out should not be used as a punishment, but is the withdrawal of a privilege (social contact). It should:

- be administered in a 'matter-of-fact' manner, avoiding angry or pejorative language and behaviour

- be administered as swiftly as possible after the undesired social behaviour; delay results in the child being unclear why he or she has been removed, with resentment and reduced effectiveness

- be brief – as a rule of thumb, use a time period as long in minutes as the child is old (e.g. five minutes for a five-year-old); prolonged use results in the same unwanted effects as delayed use

- not inadvertently include any rewards – should avoid giving the child undue attention, or using an area with toys

Table 13.1 Glossary of common techniques or procedures

Chaining	A planned programme for the reward of sequential components of a desired behaviour in stages, e.g. used in soiling to reward sitting on toilet, followed by longer intervals there, followed by depositing faeces there.
Desensitisation	Repeated exposure to an aversive stimulus while using techniques to maintain a relaxed state.
Differential reinforcement	The simultaneous reward of desired behaviour and extinction of undesired behaviour; also used when the same behaviour may be desired in one setting but not another.
Extinction	Withholding what was previously rewarding for an undesired behaviour.
Graded exposure	A planned programme of desensitisation to a series of increasingly aversive stimuli, based on a hierarchy of such stimuli generated by the young person/carer.
Modelling	The demonstration of desired behaviour for the child to imitate.
Negative reinforcement	Removal of an aversive stimulus after a desired behaviour.
Overcorrection	Change in frequency of behaviour beyond the required threshold – arguably beneficial in disruptive behaviour and adjunct to treatment of enuresis by including additional fluid load in final stage of programme.
Positive reinforcement	Presentation of a positive stimulus after a desired behaviour (reward).
Progress charts	Charts used to monitor progress, e.g. a star chart where the star is used as a form of reward.
Response-cost	Withdrawal of reinforcers in proportion to the degree of severity of the undesired behaviour, i.e. a graded extinction.
Time out	The planned brief withdrawal of a reinforcement (commonly social contact) following an undesired behaviour, i.e. an example of extinction and not to be confused with seclusion (the removal of a person for reasons of safety or punishment).

- be timed and controlled by the adult, not the child, for example by the use of a clock or egg-timer; avoid assigning responsibility to the child – 'come back when you've quietened down'

- be immediately reinstated if antisocial behaviour persists.

Rewards (positive reinforcements) need not be expensive or difficult to achieve. They:

- commonly include adult attention or praise

- should be consistent

- should be appreciated by the child, which entails adapting them to the child's individual interests with a degree of variety.

Desensitisation should always entail the involvement of the young person in its design and implementation. It should:

- have agreed, definable and achievable goals

- always begin with the least anxiety-provoking stimulus from the hierarchy of situations drawn up by the young person/carer – trying to jump ahead is like trying to jump several rungs of a ladder

- entail remaining in the anxiety-provoking situation at the time of each exposure until the child's anxiety has fallen to a comfortable or tolerable level and not after a predetermined interval; the latter may result in withdrawing prematurely from the stimulus, which results in rewarding avoidance by the resultant fall in anxiety

- always be monitored at each stage.

Star charts are commonly used as a means of rewarding desired behaviour in young children. They should:

- not be imposed on the child without age-appropriate explanation

- be 'owned' by the young person, who should be involved in their design and construction

- not include a 'negative' symbol for undesired behaviour

- be used for achievable goals, for example rewarding the absence of a disruptive behaviour is better achieved by breaking the day into three shorter periods

- be used for discrete and definable goals, for example a star for 'not hitting' rather than 'being good'

- be carefully designed not to reward undesired behaviour inadvertently, for example stars for 'not soiling' may result in the child not opening their bowels, leading to further problems – the reward should be for appropriately using the toilet

- be accompanied by plenty of praise and positive comment.

SOME COMMON PITFALLS TO AVOID

Focusing on the behavioural treatment to the exclusion of other factors may lead to ineffectual implementation. This may be due to:

- non-compliance if the family have other more pressing concerns

- an inconsistent approach by parents, which can be due to reduced communication, comprehension, ability or motivation

- failure by the professional to recognise beliefs held by the family that may block successful implementation (such as 'he's just like his father', 'she is evil because she was born too early')

- failure by the professional to recognise potential barriers to implementation, such as parental physical or mental ill health

- parents being unable to distinguish between styles of behaviour management, such as confusing 'firm' with 'harsh'

- emotional responses by parents that impede implementation, such as guilt, anxiety, anger

- failure by the professional to make a full assessment and therefore failure to develop a comprehensive management package, which in addition to behavioural treatment might need to include medication or other therapies

- failure to take into account the young person's temperament, skills, interests, motivation and ability to implement this aspect of the treatment.

Anxiety management

Anxiety management is not based on behavioural techniques alone, but is included here to be comprehensive. It consists usually of three main components, each of which can be delivered to the young person, parents or both. They may be delivered individually, or sometimes more effectively as a group therapy.

- The first component is education about the disorder, or 'psychoeducation'. This includes a description of the normal physiology and psychology of anxiety and guiding the parents and young person to relate this to the symptoms experienced, and to identify the maladaptive patterns that have developed.

- The second component comprises methods of inducing physical relaxation, which includes progressive muscular relaxation (focusing sequentially on relaxing muscles in an 'outward' direction from the head down) and controlled breathing exercises. These should be practised – by the child alone, or with a parent – at times when the young person is least stressed, so that they can be used more effectively in anxiety-provoking situations.

- The third component aims to achieve mental relaxation using techniques such as guided imagery, during which the child focuses on a previously agreed visual image or memory of a favourite comfortable, safe, but non-stimulating environment.

These techniques should be explained and experienced first with the professional and then practised at home. The degree to which each component is applied depends on the child's needs and presenting problem, and will usually accompany specific behavioural and cognitive interventions.

Cognitive therapy

Cognitive interventions attempt to induce change by influencing thinking. Cognitive therapy has been successfully used in three disorders in young people, mostly in adolescence, but with some effect in children: aggression, anxiety disorders and depression. There is some support for its use in ADHD, eating disorders and others, but these are not discussed here.

Cognitive therapy implies an exclusive focus on cognitive processes. However, its application necessarily requires the integration of social, emotional and behavioural aspects with cognition. Most cognitive therapy is undertaken on an individual basis, but can also be effectively delivered in therapeutic groups and family settings. The techniques used broadly follow three steps:

- identify distorted conceptualisations

- test the reality of the assumptions made

- correct the cognitive distortion.

These distortions to thinking usually occur automatically and are maladaptive. Such automatic negative thoughts result from an underlying view or belief (schema).

Cognitive therapy for aggression

Aggressive adolescents differ from their non-aggressive peers in that they:

- recall higher rates of hostile cues in social situations

- attend to fewer cues when interpreting others' behaviour

- are more likely to attribute hostile intent to ambiguous behaviour of others

- under-perceive their own level of aggressiveness

- generate fewer verbal, assertive responses to conflict

- are more likely to perceive aggression as resulting in a positive outcome, and in enhanced self-esteem

- are less likely to perceive aggression as resulting in suffering for the victim.

Such cognitive distortions and consequent maladaptive social behaviour reflect differences in information processing (see Chapter 4) and can be addressed using social problem-solving approaches that include:

- self-monitoring, such as diary keeping of cognitions, behaviour and affect

- self-instruction, such as 'stop–think–do–review'

- perspective-taking, to be more aware of the variety of non-hostile cues

- affect-labelling, to assign meaning to heightened arousal

- relaxation.

Significant reductions in aggression have been reported in the use of these techniques in adolescents, particularly in combination with interpersonal therapies and problem-solving skills training, with maintenance of this effect at one-year follow-up.

Cognitive therapy for anxiety disorders

The cognitive distortions associated with anxiety in childhood and adolescence are mostly assumed from empirical work, the only definitive findings relate to thoughts of being threatened or negatively evaluated by others, and negative self-reference in a non-clinical population with high anxiety, for example statements such as 'I'm going to fail'. However, interventions have been successful with up to 50 per cent response (Kendall *et al.* 1992), and usually include a combination of:

- reappraisal of physical symptoms of anxiety – recognising that anxiety has affective, cognitive and physical components together (e.g. 'I'm feeling sick again – that means I'm anxious about something')

- self-instruction in combination with behavioural change (e.g. to treat avoidance in phobias)

- self-evaluation – re-evaluate perceived weaknesses and recognise strengths

- thought-prevention

- guided imagery, using imagined or remembered comfortable situations
- relaxation during exposure to anxiety-provoking stimulus.

Children are more amenable to using self-talk than adults, which probably reflects their use of it in play and problem solving. This may, therefore, explain why this is a particularly useful technique in young children.

Cognitive therapy for depression

Young people with depression demonstrate the same systematic negative cognitions identified in depressed adults: negative views of themselves, the world and the future. These include:

- distorted attributions, such as perceptions that events are more likely to be due to external causes
- low self-esteem, such as perceived poor academic performance
- distorted perception of past and present events.

These are mediated by cognitive processes of over-generalisation, catastrophisation (the prediction of a catastrophic result to an event or thought), selective attention to negative events and incorrectly taking personal responsibility for them. Successful interventions include:

- enhancing social skills
- developing greater self-control of cognitive processes, such as punishing self less, more self-praise, adopting less perfectionistic goals
- cognitive restructuring, such as challenging the assumed evidence supporting cognitive distortions.

The impact of cognitive therapy in depression is more variable, with again approximately a 50 per cent response to treatment (Lewinsohn *et al.* 1990), which is greater than the effect of medication. One-half of responders relapse within one year, and there are no long-term follow-up studies.

Parenting programmes

There is a plethora of parenting programmes, which vary in style, structure and content but are usually specialised modifications of behavioural therapy. The evidence for the use of most is unclear. However, there is some evidence that properly trained non-mental health specialists can effectively deliver parenting programmes. Those undertaken by specialist services may be outpatient or day-patient based. The latter allows for more intensive support. The programmes can be undertaken with couples or with groups of parents. Programmes should consider how parents manage their child's behaviour and meet their child's emotional needs. It may be useful to develop local links to receive support from specialist services.

The rationale behind parenting programmes is an understanding that a child is being presented as having behavioural problems and that on assessment these are identified as parenting issues. It is important that the parents themselves decide on the priorities and rules for their family. The professional's role is to facilitate the parental implementation of these ideas (unless this raises child protection issues). Parents can sometimes request you tell them what needs doing, and whilst discussing principles with them and offering suggestions are both appropriate, it is inappropriate to over-direct them. This would not allow them to resolve the issues within the family and does not empower them to build their own skills. There are several issues that need to be addressed when considering parenting:

- The first issue is about establishing clarity of expectations and roles. This may involve exploring parental experiences during their own childhood. Parents who experienced very controlling parents may go to the other extreme and be reluctant to exercise any limits or boundaries on their own children. Parents need to be aware of the difficulties this creates for the child. Those who have very different perspectives may find themselves contradicting each other, leaving the child baffled as to what is expected of them.

- Parents may also need permission to be firm (and this may need to be differentiated from harsh).

- Parents need to ensure that their approach towards children is clear and consistent. Parents may find that they are undermined by other family members and may need to find strategies to handle this. This may be particularly true when the parents are separated. In these situations it is helpful to see the parents together. If they find this prospect too difficult, it may be appropriate to see them separately and ensure both are given the same message. It is also worth asking parents to consider the messages the child is receiving and the position they are put in if there is ongoing hostility and acrimony between the parents.

- Establishing who is in charge is important, as is improving the relationship between the parents and child.

- If a child has presented with difficult behaviour, it can very easily become a defined role for that child – the child does not behave in the required way, so the child is never expected to do so, and ultimately the child will rarely do so. Parents need to take the lead in breaking the negative cycles, and a helpful way of doing this is to focus on the positives. Rewards should also be realistic and age-appropriate, and set at realistic and achievable timescales. Asking a three-year-old child to wait a week for a reward is unrealistic. Delaying dealing with undesired behaviour in young children is unhelpful, as they will often have forgotten what the behaviour was.

- Rather than punishing undesired behaviour, desired behaviour is rewarded. This is not the same as ignoring bad behaviour altogether, but is focusing on the positives. It also enables the child to move away from their assigned role within a family.

- It is also important to be explicit and specific with children about expectations. Asking a child to be good or not be bad can be very difficult for the child to understand. What might be perceived as being good one day may be perceived as not good on another day. It is more helpful to say exactly what is expected, for example the child might be requested not to swear or hit people or to eat their meal. These are very specific and clear, whereas saying the child needs to 'be good' could be interpreted differently by each member of the family in what was expected.

- Parents also need to be aware of developmental appropriateness and be realistic about their expectations.

- It is also important that parents select the issues that warrant concern and learn to let less major issues pass. It can also be helpful for the parents to learn the child's strengths and work on those and find ways of spending time with their child that is enjoyable. Parenting is not much fun for parents if they are constantly finding themselves being negative, nor is it much fun for the child. It is important not to let the behaviour define the child and become overcritical.

Counselling

The term 'counselling' has come to be used so liberally that people can often be unclear as to what it means and who should be providing such treatments. Essentially counselling can vary from support and advice provided by informally trained staff to therapy provided by highly skilled and qualified staff, and everything in between.

There can sometimes be an assumption that all young people need counselling if they have had certain experiences, such as abuse or parental separation. It is important to recognise that for most of these experiences young people do not necessarily require counselling. Often it is sufficient if the adults around them provide enough support and have an understanding of what the young person has or is experiencing. The perceived need for young people to be counselled can be a reflection of the uncertainties of the adults involved. The problem with automatically suggesting counselling is that it can deprive the young person of an opportunity to deal with experiences appropriately, and can thereby inappropriately focus the problem on them.

There will, however, be some young people who do require intervention, and it can be difficult to identify these young people and their needs. If the counsellor is one of several professionals involved with the young person, they should ensure that they do not work in isolation. It is also important that the young person is agreeable to counselling. If a young person is insistent they do not wish to have counselling, their view should be respected. However, one can still work with the young person, perhaps, for instance, working with him or her to explore other options or ways to manage difficulties. Young people under 16 years of age should be given confidentiality, but this has to be limited by the need to disclose information relating to safety and child protection issues. It is inappropriate for a non-specialist counsellor to continue working with a young person who is deliberately self-harming or has a major mental health disorder. The primary care staff in these circumstances are probably best to focus on trying to encourage the young person to access appropriate specialist help. Primary care staff should set clear boundaries and ensure that they do not find themselves out of their depth or that the young person becomes dependent on them.

Counselling can provide the young person with an opportunity to explore their feelings and address them in ways that they find comfortable, but which are also acceptable in a wider context. Counselling should aim to improve the young person's ability to manage distress and difficult or potentially difficult situations. It can be an opportunity to enable the young person safely to explore different options. Depending on the skills, training and experience of the counsellor, several different types of techniques may be usefully employed.

Solution-focused brief therapy

De Shazer and the team at the Brief Therapy Centre in Milwaukee developed solution-focused brief therapy in the early 1980s (Evan, Iveson and Ratner 1999). It was created as a brief model of therapy that uses concepts of solution-focused thinking. The term *client* is used as the model can be used with young people and their parents.

The central premise of solution-focused brief therapy is that during conversations there will be a shift from problem-domination to solution-orientation, thus enabling development in the client. This approach can produce results for the client within a few sessions.

Solution–focused brief therapy and its application to practice

Although the approach was intended, initially, for use as a therapy, the techniques can be utilised in many situations. Elements of the approach can be practised in conversations with young people and their parents and in work with other professionals. The approach has a number of basic assumptions:

- Attempts to comprehend the origins or causes of a problem are not necessarily a step towards its resolution. Sometimes discussing the problem can be unhelpful to developing any useful solutions.

- Successful work depends on knowing what the client wants to achieve. Once this has been established, then the aim of the approach is to find the quickest and most effective way of achieving the defined goals.

- Even if a problem seems not to have a resolution there are always times when the client can find a solution. The most efficient use of time here is establishing 'what works' and building upon it.

- The client will be able to ascertain when the problem has been resolved; sometimes small changes identified within the session can set in motion a solution to the problem, or indeed lead the system to change in other areas.

Elements of practice

The elements informing the basis of practice include:

1. **Establishing a context for the work**

   The therapy is a collaborative approach to which the client brings knowledge of the issues and what they would like to change. Pay attention to what has been useful in the past and how both parties will know when the process is working and what is the preferred approach for the client.

2. **Identifying a preferred future**

   Goal setting is central to the process. It is paramount for these to be described and explored in detail, as the therapist has no separate goal for the work other than those defined by the client.

3. **Defining progress**

   The key consideration when looking at preferred future is for the client to define when they feel their work will be progressing.

   The initial focus will concentrate on when the client will know that the session has been useful. Ways of achieving this include getting the client to know what it would take to convince them that the work had been useful or by asking what would be different. It can sometimes be useful to ask the client 'third person perspectives', for example 'What would your parents see happening if this work has been successful?' It is also important to get the client to notice or identify when small changes are being made or the identified area for change is moving forward.

4. Establishing what is working

Here the approach is to focus on what is working, either for the client or those around them, rather than focusing on what elements the client should be reducing. It is vital to encourage identification of what they could be doing more of. This involves discussing signs of progress.

5. Scaling questions

Scaling questions can be useful in allowing the client to develop a clear focus on how far they have progressed towards meeting their goals. They also allow for integration of differences in perspective between the client and their family or friends. The following types of questions can be useful:

- On a scale of 1 to 10, 10 representing the achievement of your goals and 1 being no progress, where do you feel you are?

- So what tells you things are at…and not at 1?

- What tells you things have moved to that point?

Scaling questions can help the client to look at things like confidence and progress.

6. Identifying resources and determining a context of competence

This focuses the client on determining what is available to them in order to achieve goals; it is also important to identify the qualities they have, thus developing a context of resourcefulness and openness to change.

7. Constructive feedback

The effects of the therapeutic conversation can be amplified by giving feedback on the qualities of the client and the useful aspects of the process that has taken place during the session. It is always useful at the end of the session to see if the client needs follow-up or whether they are satisfied with the outcomes.

Motivational interviewing

Miller developed the framework for motivational interviewing in the context of addressing problem substance use. It is grounded in client-centred principles and is both practical and effective (Miller and Rollnick 1991). Its use in treatment for substance misuse is widespread; however, it can be applied in a diverse range of contexts when the young person needs to make changes in their life. There are five recognised phases of the readiness for change model and people may move back and forth between the phases.

- *Precontemplation phase* – the user does not see their substance use as a problem, although others might.

- *Contemplation phase* – the user begins to recognise they have problems but may be unsure and ambivalent about whether change is required and how to bring about change.

- *Action stage* – the user plans and implements change.

- *Maintenance stage* – the user applies their skills to maintain the change.

- *Relapse* – substance use is resumed. This stage may be short or long before the user returns to one of the above stages.

There are five key principles:

- **Express empathy**
Rationale behind this is that acceptance facilitates change.
Skilful reflective listening is fundamental.
Ambivalence is normal.

- **Develop discrepancy**
The client needs to be aware of the consequences of their behaviour.

A discrepancy between present behaviour and important goals will motivate change.

The grounds for change should come from the client and not the professional, although it is appropriate for the professional to suggest strategies.

- **Avoid arguments**

Arguments are counterproductive.

Resistance by the client indicates a need for the professional to review their strategies.

Labelling of resistance is of little help.

- **Roll with resistance**

Perceptions can be shifted.

New perspectives should not be imposed.

The client is a valuable resource in finding solutions to problems.

- **Support self-efficacy**

Belief in the possibility of change is an important motivator.

The client is responsible for choosing and carrying out personal change.

There is hope in the range of alternative approaches available. It is useful to prepare a 'decisions balance sheet' with the client using the above framework. There are six key steps:

- **Step 1**

Assess readiness for change by the following types of questions (in which smoking is used as an example of a behaviour that is to be changed):

Have you ever thought about stopping smoking?

Have you ever stopped smoking before?

Where are you in terms of your smoking? Are you interested in stopping smoking?

What would come to mind if you thought about stopping smoking?

Do you have any reason why you might want to stop smoking at some point?

- **Step 2**

Provide a stage-specific rationale for doing a decisions balance:

Precontemplation

'So at this point you really don't feel like your smoking is a problem for you? Is it okay if I ask a little more about your smoking so I can understand why you don't think it's a problem?'

Contemplation

'So you're saying you have some concerns about your smoking but not sure yet whether you want to do something about that. Can I just ask a little more about that as that may help you decide when you might be ready to make that decision for yourself?'

Determination

'It sounds like you are really determined to do something about your smoking. Can we discuss your smoking, as it may help us think about where we go next?'

- **Step 3**

Restate your position that whatever they decide to do at this point, you will honour the decision. Acknowledge their autonomy.

- **Step 4**

Ask the following four questions:

What do you like about smoking?

(Reflect each response and then ask what else do you like about smoking.)

What are some not-so-good things about smoking?

(Again reflect and then ask what else.)

What concerns do you have about stopping smoking?

(Again reflect and ask what else.)

What would be the benefit of stopping smoking?

(Again reflect and ask what else.)

- **Step 5**

Summarise the pros and cons of not changing versus changing their behaviour.

- **Step 6**

Explicitly leave the door open for further contact or discussion.

It can be very useful to draw up a table of the decision balance outcome as shown by Figure 13.2.

Current benefits	Current concerns
Relaxes me	Costs me too much money
Change concerns	**Change benefits**
Hard to give up because all my friends smoke	Would give me more money to spend on other things

Figure 13.2 Decision balance table

References

Evan, G., Iveson, C. and Ratner, H. (1999) *Problem to Solution: Brief Therapy with Individuals and Families* (revised and expanded edition). London: BT Press.

Kendall, P.C., Chansky, T.E., Kane, M., Kim, R. *et al.* (1992) *Anxiety Disorders in Youth: Cognitive-behavioural Interventions*. Needham, MA: Allyn and Bacon.

Lewinsohn, P.M., Clarke, G.N., Hops, H. and Andrews, J. (1990) 'Cognitive-behavioural treatment for depressed adolescents.' *Behaviour Therapy 21*, 385–401.

Miller, W.R. and Rollnick, S. (1991) *Motivational Interviewing: Preparing People to Change Addictive Behaviour*. New York: Guilford Press.

Further reading

Graham, P. (1998) *Cognitive Behaviour Therapy for Children and Families*. Cambridge: Cambridge University Press.

Green, C. (2000) *Beyond Toddlerdom: Keeping Five- to Twelve-Year-Olds on the Rails*. London: Vermilion.

Hartley-Brewer, E. (1994) *Positive Parenting: Raising Children with Self-esteem*. London: Vermilion.

Herbert, M. (1994) 'Behavioural methods.' In M. Rutter, E. Taylor and L. Hersor (eds) *Child and Adolescent Psychiatry: Modern Approaches* (3rd edition). Oxford: Blackwell Scientific Publications.

Herbert, M. (1996) *Parent, Adolescent and Child Training Skill Series*. Leicester: BPS Books.

Morris, R.J. and Kratochwill, T.R. (1983) *Treating Children's Fears and Phobias: A Behavioural Approach*. New York: Pergamon Press.

Pearce, J. (1989) *Tantrums and Tempers*. Wellingborough: Thorsons.

CHAPTER 14

Specialist Treatment Strategies

Interpersonal and other therapies
Range of therapies

Therapies directed at increasing understanding, self-awareness or insight are commonly referred to as the 'talking therapies', because they largely rely on the verbal medium. However, verbal communication can be limiting, irrespective of the person's verbal ability. Additional 'vehicles' for achieving this goal, such as drama and music, are used increasingly across the lifespan. Together with play, drawing and story-telling, they are regularly used in therapy with young people, who are possibly more open to such interventions, or may not have the requisite verbal skills (e.g. children with learning disability). Insight-directed therapies assist young people in addressing personal issues in the context of social relationships. They can enhance *understanding*, but do not necessarily provide *explanation*. Such therapies can be used in group or family settings as well as individually.

Evaluation of therapy

Many of the changes that take place during therapy may not be 'outwardly measurable', that is they may be other than symptomatic, behavioural or dysfunctional. Evaluation of the impact of such therapies is currently hotly debated. Some are more readily evaluated then others. Opinions range from using traditional experimental designs to not assessing (some of) these therapies for ethical reasons or because of pragmatic difficulties in making very individual subjective measures of internal change that are not readily compared. Research on the effectiveness of therapy is particularly dogged by issues of which specific therapy benefits which person or problem best, 'dosage' (i.e. frequency, intensity and duration) and choice of outcome measures (Durlak *et al.* 1995; Hendren 1993; Weisz *et al.* 1995).

Setting up therapy

A trained therapist should first assess a young person who is considered potentially to benefit from such therapy. The assessment will be of the young person and the context of the therapy. This should include assessing the young person's ability to make use of the therapy, identifying goals of treatment, and assessing the support available to the child by family or other support networks during therapy. It may entail a short series of assessment sessions. The young person and parents should understand the reasons for therapy (at an age-appropriate level) and what it will entail, particularly around issues of confidentiality (as discussed in Chapter 3). It is important to be sensitive to the fact that, unlike adults, a young person may not have initiated the therapy, or fully understood the reasons for it. Young people also do not have the same control over their lives as adults, and so may have limited opportunity to apply the psychological work they have done in therapy.

A plan for the delivery of therapy should then be established and agreed, with regular reviews, particularly for therapy that may span several months or more than a year, although most interventions do not need to be long-term. For most therapies, the length of each session, frequency, and time in the week of a series of sessions is agreed. These are with the same therapist in the same room. This is protected time, providing a boundary between therapy and the rest of the young person's life. Parents may also be seen at regular intervals to discuss the 'mechanics' of the therapy, but not to relate the private and confidential content of therapy sessions. They should be involved in the review meetings. Shorter-term therapy may have one review on completion. The nature of follow-up, if needed, should be discussed towards the closure of therapy. These issues remain the same for therapy delivered in the group or family setting.

Interpersonal psychotherapy (IPT)

IPT is based on the principle that most emotional disorders, particularly depression for which it was originally developed, occur in an interpersonal context, that is the person's mood disorder is intimately associated with their current relationships. IPT is used with non-psychotic patients usually in an outpatient setting, and may be used together with other interventions such as medication. It is delivered as a brief (12–16 session), weekly therapy and has demonstrable efficacy in depression in young people (Mufson *et al.* 1999; Stark *et al.* 1999).

There are two broad goals of IPT for the individual patient: education about the depression (i.e. symptoms, effect on function, treatment and prognosis) and enhanced understanding of the depression in the interpersonal context. The latter originally included focusing on one of four common interpersonal issues associated with the onset of depression, listed here, with the addition of a fifth in young people:

- grief – other than normal bereavement

- role disputes – the patient and one or more significant others do not share the same expectations of their relationship

- role transitions – unsuccessful attempts to deal with life changes

- interpersonal deficits – poor social skills, or inadequate, non-sustaining relationships

- single-parent families – divorce and separation, death, imprisonment or prior absence of a parent.

Psychodynamic and psychoanalytic therapies

Psychodynamic and psychoanalytic therapy in young people involves using verbal and play techniques to address issues through the relationship that develops between the young person and therapist. Links are made between current and past experiences. Sigmund Freud established the current tradition of psychodynamic and psychoanalytic therapies and first described its use in a child. Many schools of psychotherapy have since developed or departed from Freudian principles to various degrees. Klein, Anna Freud, Bion, Winnicott, and Axline have largely influenced its application in young people. Early writing focused on the process and delivery of therapy.

Young people who have experienced difficulties with life events or situations that have resulted in marked distress or confusion or a mood disorder can benefit from this approach, although it is unlikely to be a front-line management strategy. Identifying which young person will specifically benefit is difficult, and the use of psychodynamic therapies is often determined by provision of resources rather than factors in the young person or presenting problems. Therapy is usually delivered individually, with regular, planned sessions.

There are dangers in the inappropriate use of psychodynamic therapies with young people in an unsettled environment (where unmitigated threats are still present, basic needs are not met, or the immediate future of the child's care is undecided), with young people who do not have the capacity to engage in the process or to withstand the potentially powerful, painful, destructive or distressing emotions that can be aroused, or where the therapist is insufficiently supervised or trained. The assessment and planning of therapy outlined above is especially important to avoid these dangers.

Play therapy

Play therapy employs the same principles as interpersonal psychotherapy or psychodynamic therapy, but using play as a medium. Although it can be particularly useful in young children and those with limited verbal skills, this does not in itself constitute a reason to use play therapy, and young people with good verbal skills should not be excluded. In play technique the child is provided with toys (including human and animal figures) and art and crafts materials. These and anything created by the child are kept safely between sessions by the therapist. The purpose of play is to provide the child with a 'vocabulary' to:

- express thoughts and feelings

- explore concepts, and conscious and subconscious fantasies

- enhance understanding.

The aim of play therapy is not to provide alternative parenting, education, an opportunity for creativity, guidance, didactic counselling, or a chance to 'let off steam'. The use of toys, play and drawing provides the child with a vast array of means of expression, which is unavailable in verbal therapy (irrespective of verbal skills). The therapist comments and interprets the child's play, making links for the child between sessions and between what he or she presents in the session and events in the rest of his or her life. The planning, delivery and cautions are the same as described in psycho-dynamic therapy above.

Music therapy

Music therapy is a specific example of the use of a non-verbal communication. It is increasingly used and researched in child mental health. Music therapy can be delivered individually or in the group setting. It involves listening to and creating music. It can provide an opportunity to enhance certain aspects of emotional, cognitive and social development, including:

- imitation skills
- turn-taking
- vocalisations
- appropriate use of gaze and visual fixing
- mutual exchange of feeling states.

Family therapy and family-based interventions

Working with families therapeutically is seen to be a core skill for mental health professionals working with young people, as the family is the main context in which most young people live their lives. Whilst its influence reduces as the young person develops, it is unusual to have a treatment plan that does not take the family into account as a significant factor. Although most workers do not have formal family therapy training, they draw on some of the key concepts to inform their work, which is one distinction between family-based work and family therapy undertaken by professionals with specialist training.

In recent years, family therapy has moved away from the notion that it is possible to make an objective diagnosis of what might be wrong with a family and apply an intervention to 'fix it'. The emphasis now is to work collaboratively alongside families to develop new perspectives, which in turn can help them find new ways of being together that provide a way out of unhelpful family patterns. This way of working takes into account the differing perspectives held by different members of the family and also the various contexts in which the family exists, enabling issues of social inequality to be considered in the work. Family therapy differs from much other psychotherapy in that its emphasis is on the individual's interactions with the outside world rather than their inner world. Within these boundaries there are many different schools of family therapy. However, they all regard the family as the key to problem resolution.

As with any of the other interventions outlined in this handbook, careful thought needs to be given to when family therapy is an appropriate treatment. Reviews of outcome studies (e.g. Carr 2000) indicate that family therapy is an effective intervention in early-onset eating disorders, depression, anxiety, psychosomatic complaints and adjustment reactions. The studies suggest that family therapy is often most effective when used as part of a multi-modal approach to a particular problem. It is important not to see family therapy as a panacea for 'difficult' families and to have a clear aim in mind when considering family therapy. Family therapy often falls at the first hurdle when there is insufficient clarity about the purpose of the sessions; prior discussion with the family and the therapist can reduce inappropriate referrals. A family-based psychoeducational approach seeks to empower families by giving them information and helping them develop practical strategies and problem-solving skills. This has been shown to be helpful across a range of difficulties, again as part of an integrated approach to a mental health problem.

Multisystemic therapy

Multisystemic therapy (MST) is an intensive community- and family-based intervention (delivered in the home and community rather than clinic) that was developed in the USA in the 1970s (Henggeler 1999). MST uses an ecological model, drawing largely from family systems theory, particularly structural and strategic family therapy principles, social learning theory, crisis intervention theory, cognitive behaviour therapy, and behavioural parent training. Intervention is across all available systems in which the young person functions, such as family, school, peer group and local community. MST is based on the premise that problem behaviours arise within systems or their interface. The delivery of MST is 'manualised' and prescriptive, the purpose of which is to retain the fidelity of the therapy.

MST is a well-validated treatment model (Kazdin and Weisz 1998). It can reduce youth re-offending (reducing long-term rates of re-arrest by 25 per cent to 70 per cent), sexual re-offending, substance use and out-of-home placements. It can offer an alternative to hospitalisation for a sub-group of young people with suicidal and homicidal ideation and behaviour, and psychosis.

Strategies to use in primary care

As well as the types of question outlined in Chapter 3 on family interviewing, a useful family therapy technique that can be used in a primary health setting is that of reframing. This is where the professional offers a different perspective on a situation, which, whilst it still fits the facts, concentrates on a family's strengths. Examples of this would be where a family member's complaints are reframed as a desire to improve a situation or where a parent's anger about an adolescent staying out overnight is reframed as concern about their safety.

The aim of reframing is to give the family the opportunity to view an impasse in a different way that may allow them to break free from an unhelpful pattern of interaction. Careful thought needs to be given about how to fit the reframe with the family's beliefs and use of language. If the reframe is presented in a way that is unacceptable to the family it will not be assimilated. However, if it is meaningful for the family it will be immediately apparent from their reaction. If the reframe does not make sense to the family or is rejected by them, it will be counterproductive to persist and the worker should put that intervention aside and consider alternative strategies. Timing of delivery is crucial: if the professional worker offers this alternative perspective too early in the session, the family will not have had time to convey their concerns and they may feel that their experiences are being dismissed.

Medication

A successful pharmacological intervention depends on:

- a thorough assessment (including history of other prescribed and non-prescribed medication)
- explanation of the reason for use to the young person and/or parents
- explanation of how long the young person will need medication for and why

- willingness to discuss other options available
- explanation of the side-effects
- baseline measures and clear goals by which progress can be measured (for which it may be useful to complete rating schedules).

Baseline investigations (height, weight, blood pressure, full blood count, etc.) may be indicated. Where a drug has a cardiotoxic profile (that is it may impact on how the heart works), an ECG (electrocardiogram, an electrical recording of heart function) may be indicated. Medication should also be appropriately supported by adjuvant treatments such as cognitive-behavioural therapy or interpersonal therapy. Rarely is medication the only component of treatment in child mental health.

Before prescribing to adolescent girls, it is important to ask whether there is the possibility of pregnancy as this will influence prescribing. There can be a great reluctance to use medication in child and adolescent mental health by young people and parents, and by professionals who hold the view that their efficacy has not been sufficiently tested. This is rarely applied to psychotherapeutic interventions, which are seen as a side-effect-free intervention. There are, however, risks of subjecting young people to any treatment that is unnecessary or inappropriate.

The most commonly used medications in child and adolescent mental health are psychostimulants (such as methylphenidate), antidepressants, anxiolytics (to manage anxiety) and antipsychotics (see Table 14.1). Non-mental health doctors are more likely to prescribe medication for sleep disorders and for behavioural control than are child psychiatrists.

Medication in preadolescent children

There is little if any justification to use medications to sedate children. Medication for sleep disorders is usually not helpful in the long term, although it may have a specific short-term role in preventing exacerbation of an acute situation by providing brief respite. The antihistamine trimeprazine (Vallergan) is commonly used as one of its side-effects is drowsiness.

Table 14.1 Summary of commonly used medications for mental health disorders in young people

Generic drug name	Indication	Comments
Psychostimulants		
Methylphenidate	ADHD	Only approved specialist should initiate treatment. Use needs careful monitoring. Comes in several different formulations – immediate release and longer lasting forms.
Dexamphetamine	ADHD	Used if methylphenidate use limited because of side-effects or not effective.
Atomoxitine	ADHD	Not usually used as a first-line intervention
Anxiolytics		
Clonazepam	Anxiety disorders, OCD	Best used as short-term therapy.
Buspirone	Anxiety (generalised), treatment of self-injurious or organic-induced aggression, and in some behaviours in young people with autism	Does not cause withdrawal reactions, memory or psychomotor impairment and has no demonstrable potential for abuse.
Antidepressants (also used for anxiety)		
SSRIs		
Fluoxetine	Depression, bulimia, OCD	Also used in social anxiety, panic disorder.
Fluvoxamine	OCD	Licensed for use in younger children with OCD.
Paroxetine	OCD, panic disorder and social phobia	Can be more sedating than the others, which may make it more appropriate where this side-effect is desired (e.g. poor sleep) and withdrawal can be a problem.
Sertraline	OCD	
Citalopram	Panic disorder	May be used as second-line treatment for depression under close specialist supervision.
Tricyclic antidepressants		Not used in depression as no efficacy in children and adolescents, high risk if taken as overdose, and many unpleasant side-effects.
Imipramine	Enuresis (bedwetting)	

Mood stabilisers

Lithium carbonate	Treatment of mania, prevention of relapse of manic-depressive psychosis	Regular blood tests required.
Carbamazepine	Second-line treatment	Particularly effective in patients with rapid cycling bipolar affective disorder.

Antipsychotics

Atypical antipsychotics		These have fewer side effects than the typical antipsychotics but weight gain and sexual dysfunction may be problematic.
Risperidone	Treatment of psychosis, schizophrenia	First-line treatment, and there are studies underway to investigate early intervention with lower doses. Minimal side-effects at maintenance doses. Licensed for use in 15-year-olds and above.
Clozapine	Treatment of resistant schizophrenia	Particularly useful in those who are resistant to treatment by other antipsychotics or who have tardive dyskinesia. However, with a 1% risk of causing leucopoenia (decrease in white blood cells), people on clozapine need at least fortnightly full blood counts.
Quetiapine	Treatment of psychosis, schizophrenia	High rates of efficacy and a low side-effect profile.
Olanzapine	Treatment of psychosis, schizophrenia	High rates of efficacy and a low side-effect profile.
Typical antipsychotics		
Chlorpromazine	Treatment of psychosis	Considerably cheaper than the atypical antipsychotics. Marked sedating effect so can be useful with violent patients. Can be given orally or injected. In young people can have marked extrapyramidal side-effects. Neuroleptic malignant syndrome is a rare but potentially fatal side-effect. Licensed for use in children and young people.
Haloperidol	Treatment of psychosis, schizophrenia	As for chlorpromazine, more likely to cause extrapyramidal side-effects. Only available as an injection. Not recommended for use in children.

Psychostimulants

The most commonly used stimulant is methylphenidate, an amphetamine, which is usually the drug treatment of choice for ADHD with a strong evidence base for its use. It is proposed that the mechanism of action increases vigilance, improving the concentration of children. It is inappropriate to use it without other treatments to manage all aspects of ADHD. Methylphenidate is effective in 70 per cent of cases of ADHD. It can have significant side-effects, so its use needs to be carefully monitored. These include insomnia, mood changes, gastrointestinal symptoms, convulsions and cardiac symptoms. Medication-free periods should be considered at 18- to 24-month periods to determine whether it is still needed, although the need for drug holidays has been questioned. Height and weight should be monitored, as there is a small theoretical possibility of growth retardation, and a full blood count taken every six months to a year. Atomoxetine is now also available and may be effective where methylphenidate has been less useful. It tends to be given as a once-only dose, and is not a controlled drug so may be appropriate for some families.

Antidepressants

This is the most commonly used type of medication in adolescents. There are several types of antidepressants and the most commonly used are the selective serotonin reuptake inhibitors (SSRIs), such as fluoxetine. There was concern that the use of antidepressant medications themselves may induce suicidal behaviour in youths. Following a thorough and comprehensive review of all the available published and unpublished controlled clinical trials of antidepressants in children and adolescents, the US Food and Drug Administration (FDA) issued a public warning in October 2004 about an increased risk of suicidal thoughts or behaviour (suicidality) in children and adolescents treated with SSRI antidepressant medications. Similar action followed in the UK and only fluoxetine is licensed for use as an antidepressant for young people under the age of 16 years. The other SSRIs remain licensed for other conditions, but may only be used off license for depression. Prescribing of antidepressants has reduced internationally since these warnings were issued, with evidence of a subsequent rise in completed suicides, presumably resulting from untreated depression. However, antidepressants are usually best prescribed by child psychiatrists or after discussion with a child psychiatrist, as depression severe enough to warrant their use should probably be managed by a specialist CAMHS.

The efficacy of antidepressants in young people is debatable and certainly adjuvant cognitive behaviour therapy, individual counselling or family work are usually essential components of overall management. One major clinical trial (Treatment for Adolescents with Depression Study Team 2004) has indicated that a combination of medication and psychotherapy is the most effective treatment for adolescents with depression. The clinical trial of 439 adolescents aged 12 to 17 with moderate depressive disorder compared four treatment groups – one that received a combination of fluoxetine and CBT, one that received fluoxetine only, one that received CBT only, and one that received a placebo only. After the first 12 weeks, 71 per cent responded to the combination treatment of fluoxetine and CBT, 61 per cent responded to the fluoxetine only treatment, 43 per cent responded to the CBT only treatment, and 35 per cent responded to the placebo treatment. It is worth noting that a comprehensive review of paediatric trials conducted between 1988 and 2006 suggested that the benefits of antidepressant medications likely outweigh their risks to children and adolescents with major depression and anxiety disorders (Bridge et al. 2007).

There is no real justification for using tricyclic antidepressants, given their side-effects and toxicity in overdose, unless there are problems with using any of the SSRIs, although imipramine may be used as part of the management of enuresis. SSRIs have slightly different side-effect profiles and affect individuals in different ways, so finding the right medication for an individual young person can be a case of trial and error. However, they can all cause sleep disturbance and should therefore be taken in the morning. Progress needs regular review, with the medication reviewed 6–8 weeks after treatment is initiated. There may be benefits to maintaining treatment after remission of symptoms as a prophylaxis against relapse. A family history and the frequency of episodes guides the use of the maintenance phase, which is usually 6–12 months duration from the time of remission. In practice, many adolescents discontinue treatment before then. Antidepressants should be tailed off gradually.

In psychotic depression, the acute psychosis should be treated first. There may be increased risk of mania with the use of antidepressants; therefore, their use should be carefully monitored. Although St John's wort is marketed as a herbal remedy and is available without prescription, its side-effect profile is similar to that of the older antidepressants and therefore needs monitoring in the same way as other medications.

Anxiolytics (anti–anxiety medication, aka minor tranquillisers)

The SSRIs can also be useful in obsessive-compulsive disorder, social phobia and panic disorder. They are the first-line choice if medication is to be used.

Buspirone has been shown to be an effective anxiolytic and has potential as an antidepressant; it may also be useful in the treatment of self-injurious or organic-induced aggression and in some behaviours in young people with autism. It does not cause withdrawal reactions, memory or psychomotor impairment and has no demonstrable potential for abuse.

Benzodiazepines (e.g. diazepam, lorazepam, clonazepam) are highly effective anxiolytic agents with a relatively rapid onset of effect. The particular characteristics of clonazepam make it a reasonable first choice. However, if using any benzodiazepines, there is a need to be aware of their side-effects, especially in children. These include sedation and behavioural disinhibition, but if they are used in the short term (that is for a few days only) there should be few withdrawal problems.

Mood stabilisers

These are used to control mania and prevent recurrences of mania and depression in bipolar affective disorder. The most commonly used medication is lithium carbonate. Levels have to be carefully and regularly monitored to ensure they are therapeutic but not so high as to cause potentially life-threatening side-effects. Sodium valproate and carbamazepine may be used when lithium cannot.

Antipsychotics (also known as neuroleptics or major tranquillisers)

Antipsychotics are used to manage acute psychosis and schizophrenia. There is a range of new atypical antipsychotics with fewer side-effects than previous (typical) antipsychotics. Atypical antipsychotics are thought to improve cognitive symptoms as well as social withdrawal and include risperidone, clozapine, olanzapine and quetiapine. Whilst they have fewer side-effects, these can still be significant, include weight gain and sexual dysfunction.

Typical antipsychotics are still widely used as they are much cheaper than the atypical group. However, as young people are particularly susceptible to the extrapyramidal side-effects (see below) of the typical group, the atypical ones are preferred. The typical ones are more likely to have been licensed for use in young people. They have a rapid effect on the symptoms of acute psychosis such as hallucinations and delusions. Typical antipsychotics include chlorpromazine, haloperidol and fluphenazine. They come in preparations suitable for daily doses or in injectable forms for depot administration (giving a steady release over several weeks).

Neuroleptic malignant syndrome is a rare but potentially fatal side-effect of antipsychotics, presenting with restlessness, muscular rigidity, pyrexia (fever), and autonomic nervous system changes (raised blood pressure, pulse and breathing, sweating). This needs urgent treatment.

Side-effects of typical antipsychotics include:

Extrapyramidal symptoms

- akinesia (slowed movement)
- akathasia (restlessness of limbs)
- tardive dyskinesia (permanent movement disorder)
- dystonia (spasms and stiffness of joints)
- Parkinsonian-type signs including tremors, shuffling gait, difficulty swallowing and lack of facial expression (mask-like face).

Anticholinergic side-effects (can be very uncomfortable)

- dry mouth
- blurred vision
- constipation
- nausea.

Cardiovascular

- hypotension (low blood pressure)
- fainting
- dizziness.

Others

- decrease in white cell count
- various rashes
- increased sensitivity to sun, and therefore increased risk of sunburn
- endocrine (hormonal) side-effects, such as weight gain, gynaecomastia (breast enlargement, which may be particularly embarrassing for adolescent boys).

The use of other psychotropics (drugs that affect the brain) should be limited to specialists in specific situations.

Electroconvulsive therapy

Electroconvulsive therapy is rarely used in the UK for young people under the age of 16. It is a very specialist treatment and should not be carried out without a thorough exploration of all relevant issues. There can be exceptional clinical circumstances such as marked dehydration as a medical complication of psychomotor retardation in severe depression, and catatonia (a stupor rarely found in schizophrenia) when ECT may be the treatment of choice.

Residential programmes

Following the acute management of a psychotic illness or withdrawal from substance use the young person may benefit from a residential inpatient programme, such as a therapeutic community. This enables them to access appropriate counselling, self-help groups and/or family therapy in a more structured, stable, consistent and perhaps also more emotionally safe environment. They may also need help integrating back into school and their local community as they may have lost contact either through their illness or admission to a residential unit. Long-term admissions to residential facilities may be disadvantageous as the young person may lose opportunities to engage in the usual activities of adolescence at the same time as their peers. However, admission may be an opportunity to begin therapeutic work that can continue in an outpatient setting.

References

Bridge, J.A., Iyengar, S., Salary, C.B., Barbe, R.P. *et al.* (2007) 'Clinical response and risk for reported suicidal ideation and suicide attempts in pediatric antidepressant treatment: A meta-analysis of randomized controlled trials.' *JAMA 2007, 297*, 1683–1696.

Carr, A. (ed.) (2000) *What Works with Children and Adolescents.* London: Routledge.

Durlak, J.A., Wells, A.M., Cotton, J.K. and Johnson, S. (1995) 'Analysis of selected methodological issues in child psychotherapy research.' *Journal of Clinical Child Psychology 24*, 2, 141–148.

Hendren, R.L. (1993) 'Adolescent psychotherapy research: A practical review.' *American Journal of Psychotherapy 47*, 3, 334–343.

Henggeler, S.W. (1999) 'Multisystemic therapy: An overview of clinical procedures, outcomes, and policy implications.' *Child Psychology and Psychiatry Review 4*, 1, 2–10.

Kazdin, A.E. and Weisz, J.R. (1998) 'Identifying and developing empirically supported child and adolescent treatments.' *Journal of Consulting and Clinical Psychology 66*, 1, 19–36.

Mufson, L., Weissman, M.M., Moreau, D. and Garfinkel, R. (1999) 'Efficacy of interpersonal psychotherapy for depressed adolescents.' *Archives of General Psychiatry 56*, 6, 573–579.

Stark, K.D., Laurent, J., Livingston, R., Boswell, J. and Swearer, S. (1999) 'Implications of research for the treatment of depressive disorders during childhood.' *Applied and Preventive Psychology 8*, 2, 79–102.

Treatment for Adolescents with Depression Study (TADS) Team (2004) 'Fluoxetine, cognitive-behavioral therapy, and their combination for adolescents with depression: Treatment for Adolescents with Depression Study (TADS) randomized controlled trial.' *Journal of the American Medical Association 292*, 7, 807–820.

Weisz, J.R., Weiss, B., Han, S.S., Granger, D.A. *et al.* (1995) 'Effects of psychotherapy with children and adolescents revisited: A meta-analysis of treatment outcome studies.' *Psychological Bulletin 117*, 3, 450–468.

Further reading

Buchanan, A. (1999) *What Works for Troubled Children? Family Support for Children with Emotional and Behavioural Problems.* London: Barnardo's.

Bunt, L. (1994) *Music Therapy: An Art Beyond Words.* London: Routledge.

Burnham, J. (1996) *Family Therapy: First Steps Towards a Systematic Approach.* London: Routledge.

Copley, B. and Forryan, B. (1997) *Therapeutic Work with Children and Young People.* London: Continuum International.

Herbert, M. (1994) 'Behavioural methods.' In M. Rutter, E. Taylor and L. Hersov (eds) *Child and Adolescent Psychiatry: Modern Approaches* (3rd edition). Oxford: Blackwell Scientific.

Hobday, A. and Ollier, K. (1998) *Creative Therapy: Activities with Children and Adolescents.* Leicester: BPS Books.

Jones, E. (1993) *Family Systems Therapy: Developments in the Milan Sytemic Therapies.* Chichester: Wiley.

Kendall, P.C. and Lochman, J. (1994) 'Cognitive-behavioural therapies.' In M. Rutter, E. Taylor and L. Hersov (eds) *Child and Adolescent Psychiatry: Modern Approaches* (3rd edition). Oxford: Blackwell Scientific.

Lane, D.A. and Miller, A. (1992) *Child and Adolescent Therapy: A Handbook.* Buckingham: Open University Press.

Martin, A., Scahill, L., Charney, D.S. and Leckman, J.F. (2003) *Pediatric Psychopharmacology: Principles and Practice.* Oxford: Oxford University Press.

Ronen, T. (1997) *Cognitive Developmental Therapy with Children.* Chichester: Wiley.

Sunderland, M. and Engleheart, P. (1993) *Draw on Your Emotions.* Bicester: Winslow Press.

Trowell, J. (1994) 'Individual and group therapy.' In M. Rutter, E. Taylor and L. Hersov (eds) *Child and Adolescent Psychiatry: Modern Approaches* (3rd edition). Oxford: Blackwell Scientific.

PART 6

Medico-legal Aspects of Child Mental Health

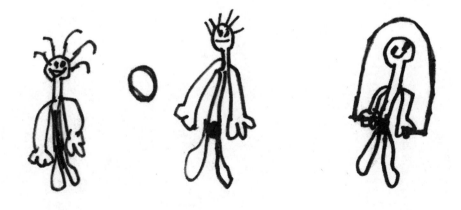

CHAPTER 15

Legal Aspects Relevant to Young People and Mental Health

The Human Rights Act 1998

The Human Rights Act (HRA) came into force on 2 October 2000 and incorporates directly into English law most of the provisions of the European Convention on Human Rights (known as Convention rights). There are 13 specific human rights 'Articles'. Some are absolute rights and others are qualified, which means that there may be situations where an infringement of rights is justified. It protects every member of society against a breach of the rights by public authorities but not by private individuals. The Act applies to all authorities undertaking functions of a public nature, including all care providers in the public sector.

The Human Rights Act and children

The HRA supports the protection of the health and welfare of young people throughout the United Kingdom. Young people are amongst the most vulnerable members of our society; the HRA puts measures in place to protect them and to improve their lives. Although the HRA is not particularly child-focused, it will affect the way in which decisions are made involving young people. Only those articles relating to young people are outlined here.

ARTICLE 3 – FREEDOM FROM TORTURE AND INHUMAN OR DEGRADING TREATMENT

Article 3 states that 'no one shall be subjected to inhuman or degrading treatment or punishment'. Legislation in the UK already protects children from abuse and harm. Article 3 raises questions regarding physical chastisement by those acting on behalf of public bodies. Although common law defends lawful chastisement or correction, degrading and harmful punishment can never be justified.

This article will also be related to complaints arising from children and young people who have been subject to restraint, seclusion or detention. To fall within this article the 'treatment' must attain a minimum level of severity, which will depend upon the circumstances of the treatment, its physical or mental effects, and the age, sex and health of the victim. This is something that those providing such methods of intervention will need to consider carefully when developing protocols and policies.

ARTICLE 5 – THE RIGHT TO LIBERTY, AND ARTICLE 6 – THE RIGHT TO A FAIR HEARING

Both articles are relevant to young people detained under a section of the Mental Health Act, the Children Act or within the youth justice system.

In terms of those young people detained under the Mental Health Act, the European Court of Human Rights has held that such detention must:

- be based on a medical opinion

- be for a mental disorder, of the kind or degree that warrants confinement

- continue only as long as the mental disorder persists

- be in accordance with the law – in the UK, the Mental Health Act.

ARTICLE 8 – THE RIGHT TO PRIVATE AND FAMILY LIFE

Article 8 guarantees the right to respect for private and family life and will have implications for children and their mental health in several areas, especially in situations of family separation or breakdown. For example, a court making a residence order in favour of one parent will need to take account of the right to family life for the child and for both parents, and consider the child's wishes. It will often strike a balance between conflicting rights, although there will not always be an obvious or easy answer.

ARTICLE 10 – FREEDOM OF EXPRESSION

Article 10 states that 'everyone has the right to freedom of expression'. This serves to encourage young people to make their views known and to impart their ideas about the services they get and what they feel would be beneficial to them. Young people's views are increasingly sought, but professionals have a duty to ensure that these views are heard and appropriately acted on.

ARTICLE 14 – FREEDOM FROM DISCRIMINATION

Article 14 states that 'the enjoyment of the rights and freedoms set forth in this Convention shall be secured without discrimination on any ground. It is every professional's duty to ensure that they employ anti-discriminatory practices in the work that they undertake with children and their families, and apply the legislation with respect to service provision for mental health problems'.

The Children Act 1989

The main principles of the Children Act are that:

- the welfare of the child is paramount
- children should be brought up and cared for within their own families wherever possible
- children should be safe and protected by effective interventions if at risk
- courts should avoid delay
- courts should only make an order if this would be better than making no order
- children should be kept informed about what happens to them and involved in decisions made about them
- parents continue to have parental responsibility for their children even when their children are no longer living with them.

Parents should be kept informed about their children and participate in decisions regarding their future. Parental responsibility is a fundamental principle and concept of the Children Act. Consequently parents with children in need should be helped to bring up their children themselves, and help should be provided as a service to the child and family.

Such help should:

- be provided in partnership with the parents

- meet identified needs

- be appropriate to the child's race, culture, religion and language

- be open to effective independent representation and complaints procedures

- draw upon effective partnerships between agencies.

Orders within the Act

The Act provides for various court orders:

- *Care Order* – places the child into the care of a local authority.

- *Supervision Order* – places the child under the supervision of Social Services or a probation officer.

- *Assessment Order* – enables the child to have an assessment but the child is not obliged to consent to the assessment.

Factors to consider when assessing the best interest of the child under the Children Act

- the child's own ascertainable wishes, feelings and views
- the child's ability to understand the treatment
- the child's potential to participate
- risk to or from the child
- views of parents and family
- implication of non-treatment (including risks to the child).

Good practice

Principles of good practice set out the context in which children's needs should be considered. These acknowledge that children and young people need to be kept fully informed about their care and treatment in an age-appropriate way. Therefore they should be encouraged to share their concerns and preferences, which should be taken into account as appropriate. Accordingly, professionals should be prepared to give people time to make decisions and consider their options (if appropriate).

Children have the right to:

- child-centred care
- be looked after appropriately without discrimination (on the basis of race, culture, gender, religion, disability or sexuality)
- develop their full potential
- be involved as appropriate in decision making (and have the right to decline involvement)
- express their opinions without fear
- receive support and information in reaching decisions
- confidentiality.

Refusal by a child whose competence may be in doubt, for example because of mental illness, leads to consideration of whether parental consent is enough, or whether the Mental Health Act (MHA) should be used. There are views that in such cases the Children Act should be used as it focuses on the wishes of the child and does not carry the stigma and sequelae of the MHA. The Children Act also expects a guardian ad litem to consider all of the relevant factors in a child's case. However, it is debatable whether the Children Act protects against possible stigmatisation and it does not have the appeal procedures inherent in the MHA.

The benefits of using the Children Act when mental illness is present include:

- focus on the child
- applicability to children who do not have a formal psychiatric diagnosis but who may benefit from intervention
- provision for a guardian ad litem to be appointed to ascertain the child's wishes and make recommendations about the child's best interests

- particular aptness for younger children (especially those under 12 years)

- perception as potentially less stigmatising than the MHA.

However, the disadvantages of using the Children Act are that it does not:

- address mental disorders

- provide specific powers to enforce treatment

- provide safeguards for the rights of detained patients

- provide for treatment without consent as it can only be used to hold a child in a place of safety.

The Mental Health Act 1983 and other legal provisions

This section outlines the use of the Mental Health Act 1983 (MHA) and other legal provisions as applied in England and Wales (but not necessarily in other parts of the UK).

Mental Health Act 1983

Parts IV and V of the MHA provide for compulsory (know as 'formal') admission and continued detention where a patient is deemed to have, or suspected of having, a mental disorder and where other criteria are met depending on the section used. The mental disorder must be specified as mental illness (this is not further defined by the MHA), psychopathic disorder, mental impairment (learning disability), or severe mental impairment. Full assessment (Section 2) and treatment (Section 3) orders require an application to be made by the nearest relative or a social worker approved under the MHA, and medical recommendation by two doctors, one of whom must be approved under the MHA. Table 15.1 summarises those sections of the MHA most likely to be used in young people. With reference to young people, the MHA:

- applies to all ages – except guardianship and after care in the community (only applies if over 16 years)

- defines *children* (minors) as aged under 18 years

- has special application for those aged 16 and 17 years.

Table 15.1 Sections of the Mental Health Act 1983 that commonly apply to young people in practice

(Details of admission and discharge procedures are not described here.)

Purpose	Section	Requirements in addition to presence of mental disorder	Powers
Assessment	2	Admission is necessary for patient's own health and safety or the protection of others	Up to 28 days admission for assessment, or assessment followed by medical treatment – not renewable
Emergency order for assessment	4	As for Section 2 (used when only one doctor is available)	Up to 72 hours admission for assessment – not renewable
Emergency detention of an informal patient	5(2)	As for Section 2 (used when only one doctor and no social worker is available)	Up to 72 hours admission for assessment – not renewable
Emergency detention of an informal patient	5(4)	As for Section 2 (used when no doctor and no social worker available (nurses holding power)	6 hours
Treatment	3	Inpatient treatment is appropriate; and the disorder is treatable*; and as for Section 2 and treatment cannot otherwise be provided	Up to 6 months admission for medical treatment – renewable

* Includes alleviation and prevention of deterioration.

Mental Health Act 2007

The Mental Health Act 2007 includes some important amendments to the Mental Health Act 1983 that relate to children and young people under the age of 18 years.

16 and 17-year-olds who do not consent to their informal admission to hospital for the treatment of mental disorder cannot be admitted to hospital for such treatment on the basis of consent from someone with parental responsibility for them.

This means that where a young person aged 16 or 17, who has the capacity to make a decision on their healthcare, decides that they do not want to consent to treatment for mental disorder, the young person cannot be admitted to hospital for that treatment unless they meet the conditions to be detained under the Mental Health Act 1983 as amended, even if a person with parental responsibility is prepared to consent.

It also means that where a young person aged 16 or 17, who has the capacity to make a decision on their healthcare, consents to being admitted to hospital for treatment for mental disorder they should be treated as an informal patient in accordance with Section 131 of the Mental Health Act 1983 as amended even if a person with parental responsibility is refusing consent. This should offer young people better safeguards.

Staff responsible for detaining a young person under the Act must ensure that they consult a person with knowledge or experience of cases involving patients under the age of 18 years. Courts who may be detaining a young person can also ask for information about the availability of hospital facilities 'designed so as to be specifically suitable for patients who have not yet attained the age of 18 years'.

'Common law'

Common law is not legislation, but a term used to describe a body of law in a country or state that is based on custom and on law court decisions. In healthcare, this has particular application where there is an expectation on professionals (and the general public) to act in another's best interests in circumstances where legislation either does not exist or cannot be implemented swiftly enough to prevent serious harm. Common law is rarely applicable in child mental health.

Guiding principles are:

- There must be a degree of urgency together with safety/protection issues.

- Intervention must end immediately when the situation is safe.

- The rights of the person being treated must be protected at all times.

For instance, a person with a suspected serious mental disorder who is aggressively disturbed and with whom it is not possible to reason may be restrained under common law if that person presents an immediate danger to themselves or others. Restraint should preserve the dignity of the person and be relaxed the moment the situation is safe. The issue for the professional is both legal and clinical: would he or she be able to defend their action or inaction in a court of law?

Admission to hospital for mental health problems

If admission to hospital is required for mental health problems the following situations may arise:

- Young people below 16 years may be admitted with consent of their parent or legal guardian. Consent of the young person is usually sought but not legally required.

- Young people may consent to admission in the absence of parental consent, providing they have the capacity to do so: parental objections are considered but normally 'will not prevail'. Whilst this applies to giving consent, young people under 16 years of age cannot refuse consent to treatment where their parents have given consent.

- If both the child and parent refuse, an order under the MHA should be considered.

- If the young person is on a care order, then the parents and local authority should negotiate (NB the local authority may restrict parents' exercise of parental responsibility if there is evidence that the parents do not act in the child's interests).

- A competent child cannot arrange to be discharged against parents' wishes: 'contrary wishes of any person who has parental responsibility will ordinarily prevail'.

INFORMAL ADMISSION OF 16- AND 17-YEAR-OLDS

This age group have the same rights as adults with respect to consent. If the young person does not consent but needs admission, consider using the MHA (parental wishes do not need to be sought, as the young person's wishes cannot be overridden by the parent's wishes (MHA 2007); however, in practice it is unlikely their views would not be sought). If the young person is incapable of giving consent, the MHA should be used above the Mental Capacity Act (2005).

FORMAL ADMISSION UNDER THE MENTAL HEALTH ACT 2007

General principles for the formal admission of all young people (below 18 years) are the same as for adults:

- The decision process is the same.

- Consider if admission or treatment is needed but refused by the young person or parent.

- If parents consent, but the young person through illness is unable to give consent, it may be in the young person's best interest to use the MHA as it provides certain safeguards.

- Keep the young person and parents informed at all times.

- Use the least restrictive intervention.

Consent to treatment: below 16 years

The issues of consent and refusal are the same as for admission (above). An additional consideration is that consent has to be separately sought for each aspect of treatment. Permission from the court may be needed if the child is neither 16 nor Gillick competent and the parents cannot be identified, are incapacitated, or are not acting in the child's best interests.

References

Home Office (1999) *Human Rights Act: How it will Help Children.* Home Office News Release, 26 January 1999.

The Mental Health Act (2007) London: Office of Public Sector Information.

Further reading

Bainham, A., with Cretney, S. (1993) *Children: The Modern Law.* Bristol: Jordan Publishing.

Black, D., Wolkind, S. and Hendricks, J.H. (1998) *Child Psychiatry and the Law* (3rd edition). London: Gaskell.

British Medical Association (2001) *Consent, Rights and Choices in Health Care for Children and Young People.* London: BMJ Books.

Department of Health and Welsh Office (1999) *Code of Practice to the Mental Health Act 1983 (Pursuant to Section 118 of the Act).* London: HMSO.

Department of Health (1989) *An Introduction to the Children Act 1989.* London: HMSO.

Hoggett, B. (1984) *Mental Health Law* (2nd edition). London: Sweet and Maxwell.

Hoggett, B. (1993) *Parents and Children: The Law of Parental Responsibility* (4th edition). London: Sweet and Maxwell.

The Mental Capacity Act (2005) London: Office of Public Sector Information.

The Mental Health Network (2007) *Maintaining the Momentum: Towards Excellent Services for Children and Young People's Mental Health.* London: The NHS Confederation.

PART 7

Exercise and Case Study Solutions

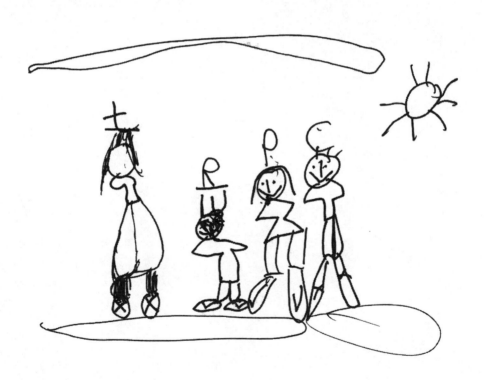

CHAPTER 16

Exercise and Case Study Solutions

Chapter 2: Meeting the mental health needs of young people
Exercise 2.3: Mapping local services

Draw up a list of local resources that you are aware of for addressing the mental health problems of young people and services for parents to enable them to parent and support young people. To your list add the problem or issue that the resource addresses, and how to contact them.

SPECIMEN ANSWERS

Services	Appropriate problems	Contact details
CAMHS	Overdoses, deliberate self-harm, depression, eating disorders, psychosis, severe anxiety, severe phobias	
School health service	Emotional and behavioural difficulties in school-age children	
Health visitors	Behaviour problems, e.g. sleep, tantrums	
Telephone information services	Help given	Contact details
Young Minds Parent Information Service	Advice to parents on concerns relating to their children's mental health	

Table continued on next page

Services	Appropriate problems	Contact details
Parentline	Advice on parenting; specialises in divorce and separation issues	
Childline	Free helpline for children or young people in trouble or danger	

Chapter 3: Assessment of young people's mental health
Exercise 3.1: Potential difficulties when interviewing young people

When the young person has difficulty in separating from parents

This is usually best managed by reassurance. It is inappropriate to insist on seeing a young child alone unless there are clear indications for doing so. The child can usually be engaged with the parent present, and the relationship built up over time.

When seeing an adolescent, it is useful to give the young person the choice. If, however, the assessment is being hindered by not seeing the young person alone, the professional can set that as a goal. Explain why it is appropriate to see the young person alone; it is usually helpful framing it in terms of development (i.e. during adolescence young people should begin taking more responsibility for themselves, and part of this is learning to present their perspectives independently from their parents).

When the parent is anxious about the interview

Clarify reasons for anxiety and address these as appropriate, for example the parent may be anxious that you are going to take their child away, criticise their parenting or give the child permission to do what they want.

When the young person is the one who makes the decisions in the family

It is useful to be clear, consistent and firm about who is in charge. It can be helpful to model appropriate strategies to the parents. Avoid becoming critical or angry with the child. It is useful to employ the strategies described in behaviour management (Chapter 13). Also, explain why the parents need to be seen separately and that they too have rights to be heard just as young people do. Courtesy and respect from professionals is due to all members of the family.

When the young person refuses to cooperate

Resist becoming impatient and be flexible in your approach. Try talking about a neutral topic, such as the young person's interests, hobbies or strengths. Acknowledge that the interview might be difficult for the young person and that they might prefer to be elsewhere. Gently try to explore their perceptions, but avoid becoming part of a game where the less the young person cooperates the more you go out of your way to accommodate them. It may seem helpful, but in the long term the young person learns inappropriate ways to engage professionals. Let the young person know why you need their cooperation.

When the young person or their parents are hostile, rude or aggressive

Set clear boundaries and rules. As a professional you do not have to tolerate abuse. Remain calm and firm. If you have any concerns for your safety, terminate the interview and rearrange to see the young person or family with a colleague.

The key principle to managing all difficult scenarios is to remain professional in your manner, which should especially be consistent and firm. There is a need to be flexible in your approach to young people and their families, but make sure that being flexible does not mean there is no consistency in your approach.

Case study: Tim (see p.51)

As a primary care worker what strategies would you employ to engage Tim?

In addition to the strategies outlined in interviewing young people, there is a need to work with other primary care staff to ensure that Tim is getting a consistent message about the importance of referral to CAMHS. Staff should avoid taking Tim on in an open-ended way as it may then be difficult to contain anxieties about Tim. It is useful to agree to see Tim for a fixed number of sessions to work up to a referral.

Case study: Samuel (see p.55)

How would you respond?

Establish if there are any concerns about what might be discussed and possible outcomes, such as making the situation worse, unclear boundaries to the meeting, potential for violence during or after the meeting. Clarify the purpose of the meeting; offer the option of the parents or individuals being seen on their own at some point in the session.

What might be a helpful intervention at this point?

Asking each member of the family in turn what they are most worried about might engage them more in the session and at the same time add to your understanding of the situation.

Chapter 4: Child and adolescent development
Case study: Sunil (see p.78)

What concerns did Sunil have, and what are the related developmental issues?

Sunil was grieving the loss of his grandparents. Their death was sudden and unexpected, he therefore had no time to prepare – there was no opportunity for anticipatory grieving. He would have a concept of the permanence of death, and the beginnings of an understanding of the beliefs associated with death in his culture. He would have to learn some of these along the way.

He was beginning to learn that death can be associated with taboo. In this instance, this is intimately related to family development, as the family suddenly found itself having to adapt to a new task.

He was also concerned that he may have caused the death of his grandparents. Children of this age can have egocentric views of the world such that they perceive events affecting them or caused by them. Beliefs originating at this age may persist beyond this phase of development, but he was able to address these in counselling.

What is the role of a specialist CAMHS in a presentation like this?

There need not be mental health problems that require direct specialist contact. Simple advice about the appropriate source of counselling would have sufficed, though an assessment was offered and this was able to exclude a serious mental health problem. CAMHS and a PCMHW can give advice about the developmental aspects of uncomplicated issues like this and determine need for specialist assessment following consultation.

Case study: Alison (see p.81)

What would you do?

Talk with her, undertake a broad assessment to try to identify if this is just a phase, whether something has happened or whether this is more serious.

What might Alison's lack of interest be related to?

Could be depression, substance misuse, some life event (parental separation, separation from a girl or boyfriend, etc.), peer relationship difficulty, having difficulty with increased educational demands, or developmental and related to issues around trying to develop a sense of self and prioritise what matters to her.

After talking to Alison, you think she is confused about her sexuality. What would you do next?

Sensitively say that it appears to you that she is unsure about some thoughts she is having (it is important to leave enough space for her to say that you may have got it wrong as she may not yet be ready to deal with the issues). If she agrees it will be helpful to create opportunity to talk further and give her contact details of local resources to help her deal with the issue. If she denies that that is the case, accept that, but then offer to meet with her again as this helps her establish you are not judging her and are open to her confusion. It may take time for young people to discuss issues relating to sexuality and sexual orientation.

Case study: Julie (see p.84)

Who should next assess Julie?

An assessment should be made of Julie's academic abilities initially by the school's special educational needs coordinator, and subsequently by an educational psychologist. She needs a developmental assessment by a community paediatrician.

What is the likely diagnosis?

Learning disability (generalised developmental delay) needs to be excluded.

Why do you think Julie's mother sought so many explanations for her difficulties?

She may have difficulty in accepting the developmental difficulties her daughter has and is looking for alternative explanations, particularly ones that may be treatable.

Why do you think Julie had so many non-specific physical ailments?

These ailments kept her off school: she may have realised that she was behind compared with her peers, and she may have been teased. Her parents colluded in keeping her off school, and may have been unable to recognise the significance of the symptoms.

What interventions would you recommend?

Educational assessment to determine whether her needs are best met in a special school or unit. Address parental anxiety about her ability, including the realities of this. Foster a positive approach to identifying and enhancing her skills, which may include activities of daily living that parents do for her.

Chapter 5: Family development
Case study: Nigel (see p.92)

What lifecycle issues, both predictable and unpredictable, can you identify and how might they be affecting Nigel and the family?

Nigel is moving towards the transition of leaving home but he is struggling with the dilemma of also wanting to stay at home to support his parents. His mother has recently experienced a transitional stage in her own life cycle: becoming a carer for her father and, to some extent, her husband. She also faces the prospect of her last child leaving home soon. Nigel's father may be struggling to adjust to his unexpected new circumstances and failing health. The family are having to deal with a range of transitions and Nigel is likely to be feeling overwhelmed by the various issues.

Chapter 6: What causes mental health problems in young people?
Case study: Leanne (see p.113)

Consider what this might be related to.

On assessment it became clear that Leanne only felt free from symptoms of anxiety when at home with her mother and was worried about leaving her mother in case she became ill again.

Chapter 8: Emotional problems
Case study: Richard (see p.126)

What should the school nurse also enquire about?

The following should be explored:

- What other worries has Richard got?
- Would he like to talk more about his grandfather and who with?
- How have other members of his family responded to his grandfather's death?
- Has anyone said anything that confirms his worries?
- How is he feeling at the moment? Mostly sad or mostly happy?
- What is his explanation for what is happening?
- Have there been times when Richard has felt down on himself or that life is not worth living or thought of harming/killing himself?
- Has he been bullied?

How should Richard's concern about telling his parents be approached?

Comment on the fact that although he says it's 'silly', he has still been able to talk with the school nurse. Ask him if a friend came to him with similar worries, what his advice would be to his friend. Explore why he would want his parents to know. Explore how they (or other family members) could support him through this. Ideally work towards Richard telling his parents, perhaps with the nurse present if he wishes.

What specific interventions should be made?

Engage him in a trusting relationship – using the skills of listening and reflecting on his comments. If there are thoughts of self-harm, engage local specialist CAMHS. Allow him time to talk through his worries, and identify ways in which Richard can reassure himself.

Case study: Tom (see p.133)

Identify the likely distorted cognitions that Tom may have.

He may:

- be hypervigilant to external cues (events and situations beyond his immediate control) and internal cues (physical features of anxiety and other thoughts of self-doubt) that suggest potential failure, and selectively exclude those that suggest success

- generalise from specific examples – for example, if he makes a common mispronunciation, he may then conclude that he is incompetent at public speaking

- catastrophise – for example, see his physical symptoms as a sign of impending serious illness, or death.

These features may all be enhanced by negative self-talk. These should not be suggested to him, but explored as possibilities.

How would you help him to identify these?

Ask Tom to describe instances when he feels anxious, what was happening before and what he was thinking or what was going through his mind. This may be assisted by keeping a diary of events, thoughts and feelings (see Chapter 13).

Case study: Jodie (see p.137)

As the school nurse, what further information might you like?

Need to get fuller understanding of Ms Mortimer's concerns as well as Jodie's school and educational history. Also need to establish developmental history and a detailed family history.

What would you do next?

Need to discuss with Ms Mortimer about the separation and its impact on Jodie without attributing blame. May be useful to explain Jodie's behaviour in the context of life events she has experienced. It is important to support Jodie and address the issues around the separation, rather than to see the unhappiness or the learning as the problem. However, it is important that Ms Mortimer's concern about Jodie's learning be addressed. It may also be important to monitor Jodie's progress, and if after the adults have addressed the issues appropriately Jodie remains unhappy or withdrawn, it would be appropriate to discuss her with a primary mental health worker, if there is one in the area, or with the local CAMHS.

Chapter 9: Behaviour problems
Case study: Jacob (see p.144)

What should the health visitor do?

Assess and clarify the situation first. Obtain specific examples of the behaviours that Jacob's mother is complaining about and explore what strategies she has used to address these. It may be useful for the health visitor to spend some time with Ms Collins explaining useful strategies for dealing with Jacob's outbursts, such as giving praise for good behaviour and using techniques like time out (see section on behaviour management in Chapter 13). Ms Collins would also benefit from putting his behaviour into perspective – she has recently had a very difficult time, and Jacob is possibly reacting to his father leaving. The health visitor could suggest some useful activities to undertake with Jacob, to enable Ms Collins to talk about his worries about the absence of his father. Some drawing exercises or play techniques may be useful, and at the same time will help Ms Collins to spend some quality time with her son.

What would you do differently if Jacob's father were still part of the family?

Would be useful to see Jacob's parents together to make sure that they do not undermine each other. It can be difficult to see separated parents together if the relationship is acrimonious, but it can help highlight that irrespective of their relationship they both remain his parents and need to work together for his benefit. It may be useful to meet them together with and without Jacob present.

Case study: Jack (see p.155)

What behavioural techniques has Jack's mother unwittingly used that have encouraged the biting?

She has used one of the most potent techniques for encouraging behaviour: intermittent reward, that is Jack on some occasions receives her approval as she is amused by it (children are keen to seek adult approval, especially that of parents), and on other occasions receives her attention, albeit shouting at him. She also models the behaviour for him.

How effective are the techniques that she has used to discourage the biting?

Shouting, slapping and repeated telling off have only short-term, if any, impact on changing behaviour.

How should this be further assessed?

Use an ABC chart as part of the functional analysis – this will give clear examples to the mother of how Jack's behaviour is shaped. This can be done in school and at home.

What is this assessment likely to demonstrate?

That there are rewards for Jack when he bites other children.

Outline an intervention to reduce the frequency of biting.

The consequences of biting other children need to be clear to Jack and to be consistent. There should be a swift withdrawal of an identified privilege following an incident of biting. Jack could also be rewarded for periods in the day when he has not bitten – say, by use of star chart and praise (i.e. positive attention).

Does Jack's grandmother have a role to play, and if so what?

Her role should be explored. If she dotes on Jack, she may be unable to accept that he behaves in this way. There is potential for members of the extended family (unwittingly) to undermine interventions. If this is the case, she should be involved in the planning, or other means of preventing her from 'blocking' should be explored.

What advice should be given to the school?

The same as given to parents. The school should be able to identify how the behaviour programme fits into school regime. Liaison with an educational psychologist may be needed.

Chapter 10: Neurodevelopmental disorders
Case study: Oliver (see p.164)

If you were Oliver's teacher, how might you approach this with the parents?

- Validate their concerns and identify the commonalities of concerns at home and school about Oliver's behaviour.

- Name those features that are related to inattention, impulsivity, and hyperactivity.

- Encourage the parents to seek an assessment of this – it is inappropriate to make a diagnosis at this stage.

Who else might you discuss this with?

The school's Head Teacher and Educational Psychologist, with parental consent.

What would be the most appropriate service to refer Oliver to?

The local child and adolescent mental health service.

Who might be best placed to make this referral?

Referral for assessment could be made through their GP or the school's Educational Psychologist.

How might you be involved in Oliver's ongoing management?

- Assessment – provision of a school report on Oliver's learning, behaviour, and social interactions; possibly completion of standardised scales about ADHD / behaviour provided by the CAMHS; facilitating any visits in the class room by CAMHS staff / Educational Psychologist.

- Ongoing management – implementation of classroom interventions aimed at facilitating schoolwork in face of ADHD symptomotology (e.g. desk location, structuring time, re-presentation of information and instructions) and addressing complications to ADHD (e.g. provision of socialisation programmes); provision of feedback on the effectiveness of interventions.

Case study: Peter (see p.169)

Peter's parents decide to chat about him with the nurse at their local Health Centre. How should the nurse advise them?

Validate their concerns.

- Make an initial assessment of development and behaviour.

- Suggest that they should discuss a referral to a specialist clinic for developmental assessment with their GP.

What form of assessment should be planned and what investigations undertaken?

- Ideally a multidisciplinary multiagency assessment comprising a full history from informants (caregivers, preschool teachers), physical and mental state examination, evaluation of functional abilities, observation in multiple settings, and communication and language assessment.

- Investigations would include: psychometric assessment, physical investigations (Electroencephalogram [EEG], vision and hearing assessments, genetic testing, and possibly metabolic tests).

What is the most likely diagnosis? A comprehensive assessment might take several months and indeed some aspects of the developmental assessment would necessarily be postponed. What could be achieved in the interim?

- Autism needs to be considered as the most likely diagnosis, along with other pervasive developmental disorders.

- An assessment of Peter's current needs and an early educational and supportive intervention package tailored to meet his individual needs does not need to be delayed while awaiting a full assessment.

Chapter 12: Mental health disorders
Case study: Tim (see p.185)

What should the management plan include?

A thorough assessment should first be made, including assessment of deliberate self-harm and suicidal ideation. In the first instance, counselling to address issues of self-esteem, social confidence, effective problem-solving and managing relationships should be undertaken. If this fails to result in early remission of symptoms, then the biological features suggest that medication is useful, and an SSRI is best prescribed. Cognitive behaviour therapy to address negative cognitions should be undertaken in conjunction with this.

Case study: Simon (see p.192)

Simon's parents come and meet with you to express their concerns. How would you manage this?

Take their concerns seriously and try to see if they can get Simon to see his GP. If there are any concerns about safety, a home visit by the GP may be the only way an assessment is possible.

After some persuasion, Simon agrees to meet with you. What are the key areas that you would need to ask Simon about?

Need to clarify whether he has any change of mood, thoughts of harm to self or others, or suicidal ideation. Check whether he has had any symptoms of psychosis and whether he is using any substances. Also, clarify whether he has had any recent stressful life events.

What roles do the school and the GP have in supporting Simon's rehabilitation?

They may be involved in ensuring he integrates back into school. Both will need to be aware of his illness and to be educated about this and about how to look out for a relapse of symptoms. They can do a lot to support Simon. The school may find it helpful to discuss with Simon whether and how he would like to handle telling his peers. Openness in the school should be encouraged but there needs to be recognition that Simon is very vulnerable and his social skills may be altered by his illness.

What cultural issues might there be?

Most Western societies treat mental illness as a taboo subject. People with mental illness often experience greater stress and less support from the wider family group than in Eastern societies.

Case study: Nasreen (see p.196)

How would you manage the situation?

As a schoolteacher, it may in the first instance be useful to talk to the school nurse or school doctor depending on their availability. If Nasreen's health is in danger, her parents need to be called to the school so the situation can be addressed urgently. Nasreen's view that nothing is wrong should not be accepted unquestioningly. Young people who have anorexia often do not acknowledge that there is a problem.

Can the school use the Mental Health Act to get Nasreen to see a mental health professional?

No. The Mental Health Act has several different legislative provisions, which can only be used by Psychiatrists, General Practitioners, and Social Workers (at time of writing) for people admitted from the community. The school should ensure that the parents are aware of all the concerns. If they feel the parents are not addressing the concerns, they should discuss the issue with the access Social Worker in the context of child protection as Nasreen may be at significant risk if she does not receive appropriate help.

What might be the specific cultural issues that need to be considered in this case?

Nasreen is likely to be a Muslim, and it is first important to check this with her. She is also likely to be of Asian origin. There may be issues if her family is traditional, in which case she may have different expectations from those of her parents about her life and how she wants to live it. Wider community issues and expectations may be more relevant. You may need to clarify relevant religious issues. But above all, avoid making assumptions and check out things you are not sure of.

Subject Index

Author Index